HOPE

FOR

HASHIMOTO'S

DR. ALEXANDER HASKELL, N.D.

© 2011

Printed in the United States of America

Published by
Advancing Medical Care, Inc.
6300 N. Sagewood Drive, Suite 421
Park City, UT 84098
866.293.1975 Fax: 866.293.1975
ISBN 1452854718 & EAN-13 9781452854717

Before making any decisions based upon the
information and recommendations found in this
book, you should first check with your own
physician. It is necessary to seek medical help in the
treatment of Hashimoto's Thyroiditis. This book is
not a substitute for quality healthcare provided by a
licensed and knowledgeable physician.

Table of Contents

Introduction   *1*

Section One   9

New Perspectives on Hashimoto's & Its Causes   9

    Insights into the World of Autoimmune   11

    Believing in Your Ability to Recover   29

    Becoming More Educated Than Your Physician   32

    Shifting Your Perspective about Hashimoto's   35

    The Primary Causes of Hashimoto's   38

    The Iodine Issue and Hashimoto's   44

    Seizing Control over the Rollercoaster Symptoms of Hashimoto's 49

    Demand the Help of a Skilled Physician   53

Section 2   59

Nine Crucial Mistakes   59

    Believing Hashimoto's is a Disease   61

    Focusing on Visualization & Psychology   63

    Relying Only on a Thyroid Prescription   65

    Thinking There's No Harm in Taking a Thyroid Medication   68

    Believing Iodine is Good for Their Thyroid   70

    The Avoidance of Iodine is for Life   75

    Using the Natural Approach by Avoiding a Thyroid Prescription 77

    Trusting their Doctors to Order the Right Lab Tests   80

    Starting with the Conventional Dose of Thyroid Medication 83

Section 3   *91*

Dedicate 3 Months to Recovering Your Health   *91*

Phase I   **93**

  Reduce Thyroid Inflammation by Lowering TSH   94

  Selecting the Best Thyroid Prescription   96

  Prescribing Incremental Doses for Hashimoto's   100

  Eliminate Iodine & Iodide   104

  Nourish the Thyroid in Preparation for Phase II   106

  Extinguish the Flame of Thyroid Inflammation   108

  Repair Thyroid Cells   111

  Kick the Gluten Habit   112

  Investigate other Causes of Symptoms   116

    Adrenal Fatigue   116

    Allergies in General   122

    Allergies to Molds   124

    Blood Sugar   129

    Candida   133

    Cholesterol & Health   142

    Chronic Infections   147

    Halogens   150

    Heavy Metals   151

    Progesterone & Estrogen   158

Phase II   **164**

  Iodine & Iodide   165

  Adjusting Thyroid Medication   169

  Monitor with Lab Tests for Antibodies & TSH   171

Phase III   **173**

    Balancing Thyroid Hormone Levels   173

Section 4   *177*

Breast Disease   *177*

    Breast & Thyroid Connection   179

        Breast Tissue   181

        NIS Channels   184

        Breast Tissue & Estrogens   187

        Iodine   188

        Iodine Research   189

        Iodine & Estrogen   191

        Thyroid Hormones   193

        Progesterone   195

        Huff...Puff...   196

        Summary   197

Section 5   *199*

Call to Action   *199*

    No One Will Ever Take Better Care of You than Yourself   201

    Know the Use of Individual Lab Tests   202

        Phase II Lab Testing   215

    Restore Your Health Day-by-Day & Step-by-Step   217

        Phase I   217

        Phase II   220

        Phase III   220

    Reflections   221

Resources   225

Prescriptions   226

Lab Testing Services   227

Storefront   228

Consultations   228

Final Words   229

Index   *233*

References   *237*

INTRODUCTION

Most people with Hashimoto's remember the time and place when they first heard this diagnosis from their physician. They were in a state of shock, wondering what had happened. What had they done and what part of their journey through life had brought them to this destination of an auto-immune disease? There had to be some answers.

With our present medical approach to the treatment of Hashimoto's, few recover. Why is this?

Some people accept their diagnosis, take their prescription and don't ask questions. Others question their diagnosis, hesitate to take their prescription and continue their journey, seeking answers and solutions.

It seems to be a matter of attitude and a sign of the times that many people are beginning to understand that our medical system has flaws and that its perspective is narrow.

In the United States, generally speaking, our educational experience is lopsided, focusing primarily on language, math, science and history, shying away from life skills and the development of human qualities such as honesty, integrity and human dignity.

Little time is devoted to self-discovery and health. Even the pre-med curriculum offers little on the subject of wellness. We memorize the parts, the body's biochemistry, and disease or pathology, all from a mechanistic point of view and really nothing about the ways of preserving and optimizing health.

We are generally ignorant about the body's miraculous abilities and because of this, when symptoms appear we anxiously seek help from our medical institutions often forfeiting our bodies, and our common sense, to a system which focuses primarily on disease and not on health.

I have heard accounts from thousands of people who recall visiting their physician, suffering from a variety of physical complaints, and after their physical exam and lab tests were told that they are fine, that everything is normal. How can this be?

Doctors are trained to look for disease or pathology, to fit signs and symptoms into a diagnosis. What we do not understand is that symptoms are the body's way of communicating to us that something we are doing or something we are being exposed to is not beneficial, not conducive to our health. Symptoms are meant to alert us, to wake us up to what it is we are doing that isn't in harmony with health.

Ever wake up with a hangover? This is a very simple example.

Certainly our medical system is insightful and scientific yet few will argue that its primary focus is on disease and not prevention. It offers a diagnosis with minimal education as to why or how the condition has come about. Seldom does the system investigate the causes for a person's illness and most often offers only a prescription which 'treats' the symptoms.

This is a mechanical or mechanistic approach, nothing artful about it. Investigating the reasons for a person's condition while offering solutions or remedies to remove or rectify them is the art of medicine. Right now the only choices our system offers are to either take the drug or to not take the drug, even though, in many cases, alternatives to prescriptions, which are based upon science and research, do exist.

The popular belief is that the doctor knows what he or she is doing and their prescription will address the condition. We are babes or infants when it comes to our 'Intelligence Quotient' about how the body works, what contributes to illness, and what supports health.

But people are waking up and using their common sense. Somewhere inside they know that their prescription doesn't really promote health.

People are searching for solutions and looking towards alternatives or a more holistic approach. They sense that health will never be found in a synthetic drug and that, just maybe, if they provide their bodies and minds with the best nutrition, plenty of rest, specific supplements and a favorable lifestyle, that they can recover their health and vitality.

And this is true for people with Hashimoto's. Their common sense tells them that there must be answers and there must be solutions.

Every person I've ever spoken to has felt frustrated with the lack of information about Hashimoto's and the minimal support and understanding they've received from their physician. If you are going through a similar experience you are not alone.

People with Hashimoto's have been dragged through years of bizarre symptoms, feeling totally out of control, without knowing why. The day their physician orders the lab test to discover Hashimoto's, they do experience some sense of relief.

"Ahhh, so I'm not crazy! There's a reason why I've felt this way."

"I have what, an autoimmune disease…and it's doing what to my thyroid? And you say there's nothing I can do…that there's no cure?"

A thyroid medication is often prescribed without any logical explanation as to why. Something about this whole scenario just doesn't make any sense.

The truth is that most physicians don't know much about Hashimoto's and have few answers if any.

But there are answers, answers that can be found in medical texts and medical journals from around the world. It's just that our system is medication oriented and there isn't a specific drug that treats or lowers thyroid antibodies. But there is a well-rounded holistic approach that does.

The "just take this pill" era is over!

People want to know what has caused their problem in the first place and then to take action and to do something about it.

We are the ones who have been living with all these bizarre symptoms which our physician couldn't explain and now we want to take control. Life is far too short to live a life like this.

We want to know why we've been given a thyroid hormone prescription.

We don't want to take a prescription for the rest of our lives unless it's absolutely necessary.

We don't want to be told what to do without a reasonable explanation.

We want to know the cause of our condition and how it developed.

If nutrition and supplements can help, we want to know about them and how to use them.

We want to know if there's anything else, any other way to improve our health which can help us to recover from Hashimoto's.

And so the search begins since our firsthand experience of the medical system has proven its impotence in treating Hashimoto's.

But where to look? Who can we trust? And where do we find the answers?

About 3 years ago I began searching for answers to Hashimoto's. For some reason I suddenly had Hashimoto's patients coming out of the walls. This became the driving force for searching for ways to reduce thyroid inflammation and thyroid antibodies. The question, or maybe I should say the quest, was to find the causes of thyroid inflammation and ways to reduce it.

I spent 3 months combing scientific and medical research putting the pieces of the puzzle together. Then I applied this research in my practice and, if people were willing to follow the guidelines, it worked.

I cannot say that everyone has recovered completely, but there are reasons why some have and others only partially. People don't feel sick only because of Hashimoto's. There are other underlying problems which are contributing to their feeling unwell which are also hampering their full recovery from Hashimoto's. This is why a well-rounded, holistic approach is essential for recovery and this approach must take into account all the causes.

Here's the first thing to think about. The full term for Hashimoto's is Hashimoto's Thyroiditis which simple means that the thyroid is inflamed. Yet a person can have thyroid inflammation without having Hashimoto's or an autoimmune condition. What is it, what are the factors that push thyroid inflammation to become autoimmune? This is just one of many questions which will soon be answered.

Nothing in this book is hearsay or lofty speculation. Every mechanism of biochemistry and every recommendation on effective ways to reduce thyroid inflammation and thyroid antibodies are referenced from medical texts and medical journals.

Your journey of search has been a long one. Congratulations! Take your time now as you read through the various sections. I have purposely simplified the content to make it easier to read, to comprehend and to put into practice.

So let's get started.

SECTION ONE

NEW PERSPECTIVES ON HASHIMOTO'S & ITS CAUSES

"It would be so nice if something made sense for a change."

Alice in *Alice in Wonderland*

Insights into the World of Autoimmune

The first step in treating Hashimoto's is to become oriented to some of the principles of health and medicine. If your desire is to successfully reduce your thyroid antibodies and to greatly improve your health you must first understand why the treatment of Hashimoto's requires a holistic approach.

Our general health is dependent upon a number of factors including the quality of our food, the purity of the air we breathe and the water we drink, and the hundreds of choices we make each day, which should ideally benefit ourselves and others.

Yet over decades and centuries we find ourselves living in toxic environments, eating inferior foods that are seldom free of additives and chemicals, and living in a society which is generally in an upheaval. We have been designed to adapt, yet these changes have happened so rapidly that millions of us are overwhelmed both biochemically and psychologically.

How does this relate to Hashimoto's and other autoimmune diseases?

Here are a few fundamental concepts about health and healing.

What is one primary difference between pharmaceutical medicine and natural medicine?

First I must clarify that in most cases the treatment of Hashimoto's does require the use of a pharmaceutical. But underlying this question is a fundamental or basic philosophy that differentiates the two. A medical philosophy, how a doctor thinks, is the lens through which they view a person and this will then dictate their approach to treatment.

Here are two models which help to illustrate.

One model uses the image of the Libran scales. Let's say that on the left side of the scale we place all that is good and beneficial for us. This side represents health and as long as the scales tip to this left side we remain well and vital. But if the scale tips to the right then symptoms or illness can present.

At birth, for most of us, the scale is tipped to the left. The heaviness or the weight of the left side is determined by the overall health of the parents, the quality of the mother's nutrition during the year before and the time of the pregnancy, the absence of ingested toxins or drugs by the mother, and her overall state of mind.

On the right side of the scale is placed all that is detrimental or harmful to our health.

And as we go through life all that is beneficial is placed on the left and all that is harmful on the right. Over our lifetime we may accumulate enough toxins and harmful materials on the right side to cause the left side to rise.

In this model when the left side of the scale begins to lift we have symptoms or dysfunction, a little discomfort or pain, a little constipation, some sleeplessness, twitching muscles, sinus congestion, allergies, an upset stomach, swelling in the feet. But when the scale fully shifts to the right we may have cellular changes, abnormal lab results, tissue damage and sometimes pathology. If you've ever played with a scale like this you know that once the scales begin to tip it doesn't take much to cause it to completely shift to one side.

Obviously, in this model the idea is to avoid what is harmful or detrimental to our health and to support and nourish our health by placing more and more on the left side (clean water & air, nutrient rich foods, exercise, relaxation, joy, love and friendship).

With this model symptoms are seen to be the body's means of communicating to us that something is out of balance, that we need more attention placed on what benefits us and to reduce or remove burdens from the right. And with this model the last thing we want to do is to place more onto the right side.

Following this model, one of the basic principles of natural medicine or naturopathy is to look to the causes of an illness (right side) and to then find ways of removing them. This doctrine goes all the way back to the father of medicine, Hippocrates, and to many other physicians including Dr. William Osler of Canada who said, "If you listen carefully to the patient they will tell you the diagnosis" which emphasizes the importance of taking a good history. A good medical history searches for causes.

Investigating a person's symptoms requires diving into their life and their habits, the quality of what they eat and drink, their exposure to environmental chemicals and toxins, to molds in their home and working environment, household cleaning materials, chronic yet silent infections, medications and their side effects, etc.

The familiar model of our modern medical system spends little time investigating the causes of a person's condition. Prescribing a medication based upon symptoms and lab results should not necessarily be the first step of treatment. For some people a prescription can be just one more thing placed on the right side of the scale.

There's another symbol or model which illustrates or explains why one person becomes ill while another does not, even though they both lead very similar lives.

We all have a sense of what it means to have a strong constitution. It's what we are born with, what's been passed along to us from healthy parents and grandparents with strong genes and a sparse family medical history.

Then there are those whose constitution is more frail, who are more susceptible to everything that comes along and who have health problems from an early age.

For this model, imagine two bowls. There's a large bowl that represents the stronger constitution and a small bowl for the weaker constitution.

Over years and decades of exposure to toxins, each bowl slowly fills. If two individuals are living in the same environment with the same lifestyles and eating habits then the smaller bowl will become full sooner than the larger bowl.

When either bowl becomes filled to the brim, any newly added toxin will symbolically cause a spilling over. This represents the beginning of symptoms or illness. This means that a person could be doing the same things every day, being exposed to the same chemicals and toxins, but one day when the bowl spills over, symptoms appear and their health or vitality begins to decline.

What is the remedy?

It is to stop any further toxins from entering the bowl and to simultaneously drain it.

This idea of drainage or cleansing is prevalent in many cultures practicing natural medicine.

How does our medical system deal with this spilling over? Most often the approach is to treat the symptoms.

How does this apply to Hashimoto's?

In 2005 the National Institute of Health (NIH) recognized over 100 autoimmune diseases afflicting 23.5 million people in the United States. Of course, this number includes only those lucky enough to get diagnosed. Many people with an autoimmune condition have been to between 6 and 8 physicians before being diagnosed. Over the past 40 years the NIH has seen the number of autoimmune diseases double and triple. Personally I've seen the incidence of Hashimoto's rise at an even faster rate probably because of the role which specific nutrient deficiencies play in its cause.

Many research scientists believe that environmental factors are the primary cause of autoimmune diseases. They certainly recognize the hereditary genetic factors (the bowl) but the key which turns these genes on is environmental (the goop in the bowl).

Some of these known factors include;

- ~ Hundreds of industrial byproducts
- ~ Chemically manufactured home and lifestyle products
- ~ Chemically processed foods
- ~ Thousands of chemicals in our soil, water and air
- ~ Pesticides, both over the counter and commercial grade
- ~ Pet products
- ~ Herbicides
- ~ Chemicals used in the industry of cosmetics
- ~ Dry cleaning fluids
- ~ Paint and paint strippers
- ~ Diesel and petrol exhaust
- ~ ChemLawn & other gardening services
- ~ Teflon and other metal cookware
- ~ Flame retardant foam in cushions and beds

You and I both have all of the above in our bodies to some degree. We've absorbed them through our lungs, our skin, and our intestines. Once inside the body, we excrete a portion and we retain the rest. Seldom is any substance completely eliminated especially if we are exposed to it on a daily basis. Each day these chemicals are placed on the right side of the scale and each day our bowl becomes a little fuller.

So what can be done?

The first and most important action you can take is to reduce as much as possible your exposure. This has to do with the choices you make each day when you walk into a market, a clothing store, the hardware store, a beauty shop, the dry cleaners, or the plant nursery.

I know this may seem obvious to many of you but people are still naïve about what is found on shelves. "Well, it just can't be harmful. Why would anyone make a product that could potentially harm us?" We often consider the effects of products upon our environment yet we are seldom aware of their effects upon our personal health. Besides, the effects are often subtle and we seldom make the connection as our bowl continues to fill.

My suggestion is to get back to the basics. Look on the shelves in natural food stores and purchase things containing the least amount of chemicals and additives. This goes for food, bathroom and household products, cosmetics, and more.

Harmful chemicals are insidious meaning they are everywhere, and most of the time they are odorless and tasteless. We seldom realize their presence. When the bowl is slowly being filled we don't really take notice of anything. It's only when the bowl becomes completely full that we start to experience symptoms. Then we begin to wonder, and the search begins.

"But I've used this hair spray for years and it never bothered me before. Maybe I've just developed an allergy to it." The truth is that the body's stores are saturated and the body is finally telling you to stop the chemical bombardment. It's crying out, "I just can't take it anymore."

Even though all chemicals and toxins are harmful, I have one primary concern when it comes to Hashimoto's. Here is an illustration of the head and neck showing the anatomy and the lymph system which runs from the top of the head down through the neck.

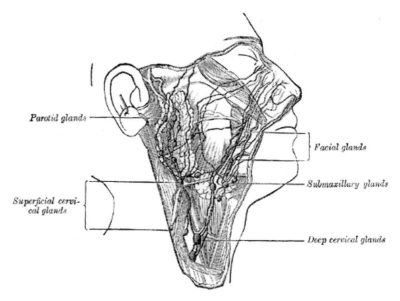

Parotid glands

Facial glands

Submaxillary glands

Superficial cervical glands

Deep cervical glands

Most of the squiggly lines are the lymph channels. There are thousands more than are shown here but these channels drain fluids away from cells and tissues from all over the head and face and even from inside the mouth and throat. These vessels run only in one direction and finally empty into the blood stream. They are kind of like the drain in the sink.

Hormones, nutrients and fluids leaving the blood stream enter areas around cells (interstitial) and are then drained away by these lymph vessels. Anything that is rubbed into the skin, put on the lips, or comes in contact with the inside of the mouth is partially absorbed into this interstitial region and finally enters these lymph channels.

Look where these lymph vessels drain. They wander into the throat, neck and the thyroid area. My major concern for Hashimoto's is the vulnerability of the thyroid to being exposed to so many of these environmental toxins because of its close proximity to thousands of head and neck lymph vessels. The thyroid is not only surrounded by lymph vessels but also sits right next to the trachea through which food, drink and the air we breathe passes.

Why are women more susceptible to Hashimoto's than men?

One factor, which you'll soon learn about, is that women have a greater need for iodine than men and a lack of iodine and iodide play major roles in the development of Hashimoto's. If you are a physician reading this last sentence don't give up on me yet. I'll show the research which explains this point.

The second factor is that women are often exposed to a greater number of chemicals from around the house and from just being a woman. They are exposed to cleaning materials, household sprays, hair dyes, nail polish and polish removers, lipsticks, facial creams, eyeliners, chemicals to straighten or curl their hair, leg and underarm hair removers, perfumes, etc., etc., etc.

One group of these chemicals is called phthalates which are known endocrine disrupting chemicals (you'll soon learn how to protect yourself from these toxins) and are found in cosmetics to make them creamier, plastics to make them more pliable, children's toys, plastic straws and more. Never sip hot drinks through a plastic straw.

These phthalates in cosmetics and lipsticks and are drawn in through the skin to find their way into the lymph to pass around and through the thyroid gland. You must completely avoid chemicals and toxins such as phthalates. You must stop adding to the bowl.

U.S. cosmetic manufacturers on the whole are still using this ingredient while European and Japanese manufacturers have banned it.

What to do?

Ideally, it is to reduce your exposure and to empty the bowl. You can also use supplements and detox formulations to mop up these chemicals and to help with their excretion. There are other means as well.

Here are a couple of personal accounts with the filling and emptying of my bowl.

I was raised on a cattle ranch and had my share of exposure to chemicals. I remember the fog bank of DDT spray to reduce the mosquito population.

I remember the barrel headed "magnum" fumigator spray apparatus used for killing spiders and other eight legged creatures.

Once or twice a year we'd fill a large tank with an herbicide used to kill weeds in the irrigation ditches in order to improve the flow of water. I usually drove the tractor and a hired hand would follow alongside the tank spraying the white milky liquid. I can still remember the smell.

We had a gardener who every week applied a variety of herbicides to our gardens. Once I drank some of this liquid out of a watering can thinking it was simply water. That was a big mistake and it was stomach pumping time.

Fortunately as far as the use of antibiotics we lived far from town, so warmed olive oil was the medication of choice for earaches after swimming. I did have a phobia about needles, and the one time they tried to stick me at the age of 6 with a syringe full of penicillin for an ear infection, they encountered the Hulk. I kicked everything that came within 3 feet. They never got to me even though a doctor and a nurse tried to hold me down. My mother told me years later that they had to repaint the room.

When I started reading about natural healing, I was introduced to some works by Upton Sinclair and Patricia Bragg on fasting. It sounded great and I was psyched up for feeling clean and light.

Well within 24 hours of drinking nothing but water I was puking by the side of the road and throwing up some of the most putrid vial fluid I'd ever seen. I thought cow pies smelled bad! After that exorcism I really and truly felt so light and clear headed. It was remarkable.

One way of emptying the bowl is by taking nothing but water. The biochemistry of what happens during a water fast is beyond the scope of this book, but there are many books available on the subject. I don't believe there is any harm in fasting for 24 hours with only one consideration when it comes to Hashimoto's, and that is the toxic stress that results from it.

As you will learn, with Hashimoto's there is often adrenal fatigue. This fatigue is mostly due to the body dealing with fluctuating thyroid hormones, exposure to environmental toxins, the lack of essential nutrients, and an immune system which is often in a state of alarm.

The adrenals make several hormones with the most important one being cortisol. You are familiar with the drug hydrocortisone being an anti-inflammatory, well hydrocortisone was designed after the adrenal hormone cortisol. It is the body's own anti-inflammatory. Having optimal levels of cortisol helps the body to keep any inflammation under control.

Thyroiditis = Thyroid Inflammation

Cortisol = Body's Anti-inflammatory

Cortisol has other important roles as well. It helps the immune system to fight infections, regulates blood sugar and increases our rate of metabolism or energy production. Fatigue can be a combination of low blood sugar, low thyroid hormones and low levels of cortisol. With low cortisol production we can have a simple cold or flu that takes weeks to recover from. If we get less than 7 hours of sleep, with low cortisol, we can feel sluggish the whole day. We can also feel easily overwhelmed. Any stress is just too much and adds to our fatigue and immune dysfunction. More about this important hormone is covered in another chapter.

Fasting is a stress upon the body because we aren't providing it with the usual food and nutrients, and because fasting triggers the release of stored toxins. When we don't eat the body must adapt. Since we require glucose to stay alive the body converts our fat into sugar or glucose, and fat cells are the primary tissue where toxins are stored. So when we fast, and fat is broken down or converted to glucose, out come the toxins.

To minimize this stress and to maximize the benefits, if you decide to do a 24 hour fast, on the day of and the day after the fast, you must be extremely low key. This means that you get to do whatever you want. Yay!!

You can lay around and play around. You can sit by the fire all day long, listen to your favorite music, enjoy hot baths with candles, read books… whatever you like. You can drink hot herbal teas as long as they are caffeine free. Lemon in water is fine as well.

There are other means of emptying the bowl. These would include detox formulations taken on an empty stomach. You might want to use these during the water fast. They can also be used first thing in the morning and then waiting for an hour before eating. Here are a few products as examples.

   ~ Metabolic Cleanse from Douglas Labs
   ~ LivDetox from Douglas (specific for liver and gall bladder)
   ~ BioCleanse Plus from Biogenesis

Another great way to cleanse is through the use of saunas and hot baths with magnesium sulfate crystals or Epsom salts. One patient with episodes of sudden disorientation and fatigue figured out that a very hot 15 to 20 minute shower would bring him rapid relief.

We finally discovered that these episodes happened on a cycle of every two weeks on Friday evenings. We thought that maybe it was the result of stress from the week but he doubted this since he enjoyed his work a lot. It turned out that Fridays were the days when their gardener would come to care for the lawn and shrubs using liberal amounts of various herbicides and sprays.

On warm summer nights, enjoying a cocktail on his beautiful patio overlooking his lush garden was when he experienced his bizarre set of symptoms.

The point is that the hot showers helped to eliminate these chemicals through his skin, enough to bring him relief. I have heard other stories from people who have been through sauna cleanses. They claimed skin color changes and strange skin odors as chemicals were being excreted. They all said that saunas helped them to feel much better both physically and mentally.

Summary

It may be that environmental toxins and chemicals are the primary cause of many autoimmune conditions. They do play their part with Hashimoto's, yet Hashimoto's is a little different from most other autoimmune conditions. Its origin is triggered by specific nutrient deficiencies which you'll soon learn about.

I have noticed that those who recover from Hashimoto's have less history of environmental exposure to toxins, have a cleaner medical history and have used fewer pharmaceuticals. Those with a more toxic history take a lot longer to improve and must engage in some form of detoxification through saunas, fasting, and cleansing supplements.

"You gain strength, courage and confidence by every experience in which you really stop to look fear in the face. You are able to say to yourself, 'I have lived through this horror. I can take the next thing that comes along.' You must do the thing you think you cannot do."

Eleanor Roosevelt

Believing in Your Ability to Recover

Almost every single person with Hashimoto's has a story. The most frequent stories include years and even decades of debilitating, mysterious, and often unexplainable symptoms. Everyone has experienced frustration, fear and confusion because no one understood them, not even their physician.

Many received a previous diagnosis of hypothyroidism and even though medicine recognizes the primary cause of hypothyroidism to be Hashimoto's, physicians seldom check for it. [1]

Finally, sometimes at their patient's request, their doctor orders labs to discover Hashimoto's, this foreign, Oriental sounding disease. This diagnosis brings some relief, for at least now they know they aren't crazy, that their symptoms are not all in their head.

Yet then they are faced with an illness that no one seems to know much about. Their doctor's explanations are vague and they are told there isn't a cure. They're handed a prescription and told it's for life.

With Hashimoto's <u>everyone</u> goes through intense periods of anxiety and feeling hopeless about their condition and about their recovery. Since there is apparently so little understanding of Hashimoto's, every person experiences some degree of despair and loneliness.

I'm here to tell you that medical research does explain the causes of Hashimoto's and how to effectively treat it. Because of this research and the improvements I've witnessed in patients, I do not categorize Hashimoto's as a disease but rather a condition which is primarily the result of nutrient deficiencies and nutritional habits.

You would be amazed at how many people have Hashimoto's and don't even know it. A recent study gathered 67 women and 62 men who had neither a personal or family history of thyroid disease. All were tested for TPO antibodies. Twenty-eight women and 28 men had positive antibody titers.[2] That's 43% of the group! This is outrageously high. There are tens of millions out there with Hashimoto's.

Your advantage is that you know you have it and soon you will learn ways to improve it. Millions of people are sick and don't know why and until they are diagnosed with Hashimoto's will go from one doctor to the next, receiving one prescription after another, with little relief and more side effects.

My sincere hope is that by passing along this information you will experience a renewed sense of hope and will rediscover the determination it takes to regain your health.

"In the long run, we shape our lives, and we shape ourselves. The process never ends until we die. And the choices we make are ultimately our own responsibility."

Eleanor Roosevelt

Becoming More Educated Than Your Physician

There's no one else in the entire world who is more motivated to take care of your health than you. For this reason you can no longer take the easy road of turning your body over to a physician and expect to get well.

The long term effects of Hashimoto's can be devastating if it's not treated. There is an abundance of excellent scientific research on Hashimoto's, about its causes, treatment, and its connection with other health matters.

So how is it that your physician doesn't know about this research even though he or she has, in our society, been placed in the position of helping you to recover from Hashimoto's?

The answer to this question is one reason why it's important to shift your relationship to your physician away from one of authority, to being another member of your team.

The duty of most physicians is to diagnose their patient through the use of the physical exam, lab testing, imaging and tissue biopsies. Once diagnosed the doctor's options are to prescribe a medication or to refer to a specialist. The selection of the prescription is based upon the guidelines of their medical board. Seldom will a physician prescribe supplements or herbs, even though articles in medical journals often highlight effective natural treatments for a wide variety of conditions.

The most common prescription for Hashimoto's is a thyroid medication, usually Synthroid or a form of Levothyroxine. Sometimes other prescriptions may be included to lessen other unfavorable symptoms of Hashimoto's.

The thyroid prescription is very, very important. I have not known of a single person that has been able to recover from Hashimoto's who didn't have to initially use this medication. But this approach is only the first step of many on the road to recovering from Hashimoto's. This single approach of prescribing a thyroid medication does not in any way address the cause of Hashimoto's nor does it improve the function or the health of the thyroid gland.

So use your doctor. He or she is an important ally in your recovery, yet do not expect them to be the authority or expert on this subject. In fact by the time you complete this book, you will know more about the science and biochemistry of Hashimoto's, and possess more practical and clinically relevant knowledge than your physician.

"The most beautiful thing we can experience is the mysterious.

It is the source of all true art and science."

Albert Einstein

Shifting Your Perspective about Hashimoto's

Our thoughts are much more powerful than we realize, so powerful that a person can actually think themselves sick. We see the power of thought when a person receives the diagnosis of a terminal disease. Something clicks inside them and they often forfeit their will and surrender to their demise.

Therefore, if a person can think themselves sick, can a person think themselves well? This is the world of psychology, of meditation and the various forms of faith healing.

Some conditions can originate primarily from a person's psyche, yet Hashimoto's, because its origin is primarily due to nutrient deficiencies and maybe secondarily to toxins, is not psychologically based. You can sit cross legged on a pillow and meditate on health for 40 hours a week and you will not get to the core of Hashimoto's. It is not a mental condition. Certainly trusting in the innate wisdom of the body for recovery is very important, yet specific nutrients are essential.

Every thought or belief, though invisible and even unconscious, becomes the chemistry that flows through our veins. This "psychochemistry" has an incredible influence upon every cell that it bathes and envelopes. It possesses an inherent power to nourish as well as to destroy.

Obviously the chemistry of hope and love is a completely different experience when compared with the chemistry of fear and hopelessness. The bodily sensations we experience under their influence are totally different.

Our psychochemistry travels deep within us, causing subtle and sometimes imperceptible effects. Many studies have demonstrated the consequences of our emotions upon the white blood cells of our immune system.

Since Hashimoto's is an autoimmune condition it is extremely important to learn how to shift our thoughts and points-of-view *about* Hashimoto's to being positive and hopeful. This helps to alter our psychochemistry which encourages our recovery.

The wonderful thing about working to improve our psychochemistry is that we know it almost immediately. When we shift an attitude or belief away from fear towards hope, we <u>know</u> it, we feel it, and we experience it firsthand.

Instinctively we all know that fears and worries are not good for us, are not leading us towards wellness. We also <u>know</u> the power of hope and inspiration and how they are allies.

With psychochemistry it's as if we have access to our own pharmacy within and what is dispensed into our bloodstream is directly related to our thoughts and beliefs.

So here's the plan for engaging your psychochemistry in the treatment of Hashimoto's.

Right now you are in limbo, a state of uncertainty, of confusion, and feeling a lack of control. You want to understand Hashimoto's and to be free of its stigma, to regain your energy, to feel emotionally stable, to have the sense of being empowered, and in control of your health again.

How we get to this end result comes first through education, which is a very stable platform upon which we will build the course of treatment.

"Opportunities don't often come along.
So, when they do, you have to grab them."

Audrey Hepburn

The Primary Causes of Hashimoto's

Knowledge is power. To fully engage the miraculous process of healing requires altering your beliefs by <u>knowing</u> what to do and <u>why</u> you are doing it. This is the reason for the rising tide in our population which no longer accepts the "just take this pill" approach from their physician.

We want to know. We want to understand. We want to take control of our health and our destiny.

So here is essentially what you need to know about Hashimoto's that will explain why it is a condition and not a disease.

TSH, or Thyroid Stimulating Hormone, is normally secreted by a gland in the brain (pituitary) when thyroid hormones in the blood are low. TSH stimulates thyroid cells to make more thyroid hormones. As thyroid hormones are produced and are increased in the blood stream, the secretion of TSH slows down.

Simple... it's a kind of "see-saw" effect. When thyroid hormones go down then TSH goes up.

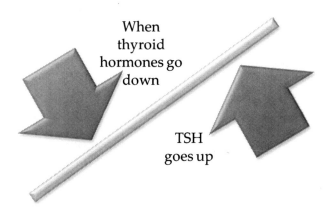

And when thyroid hormones go up then TSH goes down.

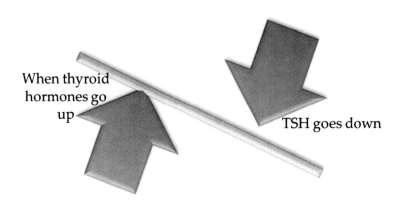

There are a number of very intricate steps taking place inside thyroid cells to make thyroid hormones. One step is preparing iodine from iodide in order to make the thyroid hormone.[3] Iodide is absorbed into the thyroid cell and must then be converted to iodine. This conversion requires hydrogen peroxide ($H2O2$) that is made within the thyroid cell. The production of hydrogen peroxide (H2O2) is stimulated by TSH. [4] [5] [6] [7] [8] This is very important to understand and bears repeating.

In order to make its hormones the thyroid needs iodine. In fact there are several thyroid hormones and each of them requires iodine to be made. No iodine, no thyroid hormones. But thyroid cells don't absorb iodine, they absorb iodide and this iodide must be changed into iodine.

This change takes place inside thyroid cells in the presence of hydrogen peroxide. When more thyroid hormones are needed, TSH stimulates thyroid cells to make more hydrogen peroxide.

So what's going to happen if there isn't enough iodide? What if a person is on a salt free diet and avoids iodized salt? Well if the thyroid doesn't get what it needs to make its hormones then thyroid hormone production declines and the person suffers from low thyroid hormones. And what happens with TSH production?

When thyroid hormones are low TSH will continue to increase in an attempt to stimulate the thyroid to make more hormones.

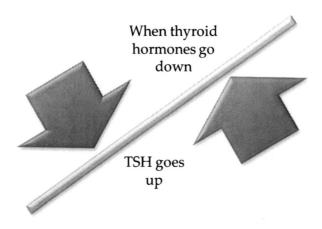

When thyroid hormones go down

TSH goes up

When there's a lack of iodide, and for that matter any nutrient the thyroid requires to make its hormones, then TSH will remain elevated. And as long as it remains elevated it will continue to stimulate thyroid cells to make hydrogen peroxide.

If this goes on for too long these thyroid cells become irritated, inflamed, and damaged by the increased hydrogen peroxide. Do you see where we are going? There are a few theories about the origins of Hashimoto's but the leading theory sees elevated TSH as being the cause of thyroid inflammation due to the increased production of hydrogen peroxide.[9]

We know that H2O2 causes oxidative *damage* and *inflammation*.[10] [11] This can harm DNA inside cells and eventually lead to thyroid cell destruction.[12] When thyroid cells destruct, H2O2 leaks into areas surrounding the thyroid, signaling white blood cells to converge on the site to begin the clean up process. These white cells are like scavengers and play an important role. Yet sometimes they become overly zealous and actually attack the ingredients of the thyroid cells including an enzyme called thyroperoxidase (thus elevated thyroperoxidase antibodies).[13]

So, is elevated TSH the root cause or reason for increased hydrogen peroxide production and inflammation? Well, yes, but what about the reasons for TSH being elevated in the first place?

The primary reason for elevated TSH is low levels of circulating thyroid hormones. Therefore, whatever the reason may be, if the thyroid cannot make optimal levels of thyroid hormones, you'll have elevated TSH. If TSH remains high for years and decades, the increased hydrogen peroxide will eventually lead to thyroid inflammation. Therefore elevated TSH is not truly the origin of thyroiditis, it's the lack of nutrients required by the thyroid to make its hormones.

The first step in reducing thyroid inflammation is to reduce TSH and the way to do this is to increase thyroid hormone levels. Then logically it would seem that all you need to do is to provide thyroid cells with the nutrients they need to produce more hormones. However, with Hashimoto's, this is not the answer and I'll explain why in just a moment.

There are several nutrients which thyroid cells require in order to make thyroid hormones and if any one of them is deficient or insufficient then it's impossible for the thyroid to produce optimal levels of thyroid hormones. So why not just give these nutrients? One of the nutrients is iodide but with Hashimoto's this important trace mineral must be avoided.

"The more that you read, the more things you will know.

The more you learn the more places you'll go."

Dr. Seuss

The Iodine Issue and Hashimoto's

There are some who believe that Hashimoto's is caused by taking iodine and iodide. Some studies have shown that in areas of the world where iodide has been supplemented there's been an increased incidence of Hashimoto's. On the surface this appears to be true, but when you understand thyroid chemistry and physiology you'll realize why this hypothesis is false.

It's important for you to know about how doctor's think because as you begin to believe in the possibility of treating and curing Hashimoto's you must avoid confusion and doubt.

So many times I've heard stories where patients have approached their physicians with an idea or theory they'd like to share or maybe a request for specific blood tests or a prescription. So often their physician's response is derogatory and condescending.

In an autoimmune condition the immune system's white blood cells are attacking normal body tissues in a state of chaos and confusion. Therefore the less confused and the more certain and educated you are, the better it is for your immune system.

Let's get back to iodine and iodide. Both these trace minerals stimulate the production of TSH and for a very important reason. I'll repeat this again. Iodine and iodide stimulate the production of TSH.[14] [15] [16] [17] In another section I'll show you lab results to prove this. From what you know about thyroid inflammation, we definitely do not want to stimulate TSH production.

Why would iodine and iodide cause an increase in TSH?

Iodine and iodide are extremely valuable to the body and the hormone TSH helps to store them in various tissues. These precious trace minerals not only play an important role in healthy metabolism and energy production, they also protect our tissues from environmental toxins known as Endocrine Disrupting Chemicals. Without iodine and iodide these chemicals have harmful effects including growths and mutations.

So why would some believe iodide and iodine to be the cause of Hashimoto's?

Since iodine and iodide increase TSH and TSH increases hydrogen peroxide production in thyroid cells, this will, to some degree, result in thyroid inflammation. Yet as long as we are eating plenty of nutritious foods we will have plenty of antioxidants to help reduce this inflammation. These antioxidants effectively quench or neutralize inflammation.

Generally speaking, people are low in antioxidants and this often leads to many health problems. Let's say that we have two individuals who are eating pretty much the same foods and they are both avoiding cholesterol foods due to cholesterol propaganda and the marketing of lipid lowering drugs. Therefore they have reduced their eggs and meat intake. Maybe they have a reduced budget due to the economy and are eating the less expensive proteins such as chicken. They tend to buy frozen foods because of convenience and cost, and fruits are eaten occasionally. Maybe they have incorporated a kind of vegetarian regime for a few nights per week. Let's say that the only difference between these two individuals is that one adds iodized (iodide) table salt while the other does not since they've heard that salt is not good and can cause high blood pressure.

Both of their diets are low in selenium. If you search "selenium foods" you'll find that animal proteins are the richest source. Selenium is the most important trace mineral for the body's production of an antioxidant called glutathione and both glutathione and selenium have the most positive research results in the treatment of Hashimoto's and the reduction of thyroid antibodies.

The person that is abstaining from iodized salt will not have the primary nutrient needed by the thyroid to make optimal thyroid hormones. This will result in an increase in TSH.

The second person having iodized salt is providing their thyroid with what it needs, yet their iodide intake will also increase TSH to some extent, enough to cause some degree of thyroid inflammation.

Because both diets are poor in selenium their ability to reduce thyroid inflammation is compromised. I believe these two scenarios are just a couple of reasons why we are seeing a tremendous increase in the number of people with Hashimoto's.

This comes back to the study published in a major medical journal called *The Lancet*. In 1975 they found that the rate of breast cancer in Japan was much, much less than the U.S.

The only difference between the 2 populations was the intake of foods containing iodine and iodide, the Japanese being much higher. We have no indication of there being a higher rate of Hashimoto's or thyroid inflammation in the Japanese population, and so the connection between increased iodide and iodine being the cause of Hashimoto's doesn't make sense.

At the same time if you look a little deeper into this study, the higher intake of iodine in the Japanese population was through food and not through iodide added to salt or iodide and iodine supplements. And their foods were also rich in selenium.

Just to be clear, we need to reduce TSH and the only way to do this is by increasing circulating thyroid hormones. But we can't do this by providing the thyroid with what it needs to make its hormones because the most important nutrient, iodide, will stimulate TSH production.

To provide the body what it needs to increase circulating thyroid hormones requires a thyroid prescription. This does not mean that a person will be taking this prescription for the rest of their life.

"It is this belief in a power larger than myself and other than myself which allows me to venture into the unknown and even the unknowable."

Maya Angelou

Seizing Control over the Rollercoaster Symptoms of Hashimoto's

There are clusters or sets of symptoms with Hashimoto's. They can be fatigue, weight gain, hair loss, apathy, low sex drive, etc. They can also include too much energy, restlessness, insomnia, with rapid heart rate and anxiety.

People with Hashimoto's can rollercoaster back and forth between these two sets of symptoms, especially in the beginning stages.

To begin with, TSH will usually be in the higher than normal range in response to low thyroid hormones. This stimulates H2O2 production and thyroid inflammation. If this goes on for years these inflamed thyroid cells will begin to break apart with the release of thyroid hormones in sudden bursts, which stimulate the hyper set of symptoms.

In the later stages, TSH can be on the low side in some people which often means that their pituitary, which makes the TSH, is fatigued and just can't make more of it.

It's been my experience that when a person with Hashimoto's has elevated TSH they are easier to treat than the person with a low TSH.

When someone is experiencing the hyper side of thyroid symptoms due to the sudden release of thyroid hormones due to thyroid cell destruction, which is basically temporary hyperthyroidism, it's very important to not make things worse by becoming emotionally engaged. There is much that can be done to minimize the intensity and duration of excess thyroid hormones.

Remember the connection between our emotional state and the activity of our white blood cells. The sooner we can move ourselves away from the hyper side the better it will be for our thyroid gland.

When you see someone blowing into a paper bag and then smashing it, your nervous system is ready for the bang. The experience is not nearly as frightening as when someone sneaks up behind you and explodes it right behind your head. When you are prepared for the bang, your nervous and endocrine systems do not over react and very quickly your blood pressure and heart rate return to normal.

With Hashimoto's, understanding the cause of the hyper symptoms, that they are simply due to the sudden release of thyroid hormones, your emotions of fear and anxiety will not be nearly as intense.

Have a plan for the next time these symptoms come on. Select some music that is relaxing or more centering and meditative. This can really foreshorten this hyper experience. Being calm will help your white cells to also become calmer.

I went through a very serious crisis a number of years ago and experienced being overwhelmed by fear and anxiety. Intellectually I knew that these emotions were not helping me at all to deal with the situation. I had received a lot of training in a type of breath work from Dr. Stan Grof. When these anxious emotions would suddenly shoot into my veins my only choice was to sit with them, to relax every muscle and to breathe deeply into the areas of my body where these emotions seemed to cling. I was amazed, and truly grateful, to see how well this intentional and conscious breathing helped to dissolve these fearful and irrational emotions.

This is true for the emotional side of the hyperthyroid symptoms of Hashimoto's as they pass through in waves. Dispelling the fearful emotions that tend to magnify the hyper symptoms will help recover your equilibrium more quickly.

There is also an important attitude here. There's a kind of centering and surrendering to the experience as it happens. You allow the body to go through the experience with the attitude that you possess a miraculous inner wisdom that can bring your body back into balance, into a state of equilibrium or homeostasis.

The posture of the mind is to surrender or to allow. The posture of the heart is the belief or the faith that *It* has the ability to return the body back to normal. And the posture of the body is one of total relaxation.

The more we can decrease the intensity of these clusters of hyperactivity the more we can improve its aftermath of fatigue, depression and just feeling wiped out. The best news is that most people have found that within a few weeks of using specific antioxidants and getting their TSH under control with the right dose of thyroid medication, that these ups and downs are much, much better.

"Unless someone like you cares a whole awful lot,

nothing is going to get better. It's not."

Dr. Seuss

Demand the Help of a Skilled Physician

Most of us experience some degree of frustration when it comes to the quality of care we receive from our physician and our medical system. We are becoming more and more disillusioned with the routine prescription in the absence of any explanation as to why we are ill.

A part of us resents being labeled without any explanation or knowledge offered as to why and what to do. Sometimes our only alternative is to search online for answers and solutions. We seek help and to regain some control over our lives and our health.

To recover from Hashimoto's requires self-motivation and determination. Even though this falls mostly upon your shoulders, you will need the help of a medical professional. Here are a few reasons why.

1. If your TSH is above 1.0 then you'll need a thyroid prescription in order to bring it down.

Because TSH stimulates thyroid cells to produce hydrogen peroxide it's obvious that TSH must be reduced.

TSH is reduced by increasing thyroid hormone levels. Since we must avoid iodine and iodide, the only option for increasing thyroid hormones is to take a thyroid hormone prescription.

I hope this is clear. Most people are already iodine and iodide insufficient and by avoiding these two trace minerals in order to lower TSH their thyroid will not be able to produce much of its own thyroid hormones. Therefore a prescription for thyroid hormones is necessary for lowering TSH.

When you swallow a thyroid medication the hormone(s) enters the blood stream and signals the pituitary to reduce its production of the hormone TSH. Therefore a physician is necessary for writing the script.

You'll soon learn more about the safe and effective use of thyroid medication.

2.   Evaluating thyroid antibody levels.

A person is unable to physically sense their antibody levels. They may be able to sense their thyroid hormone levels but not their antibodies. Sometimes a person will have sensations in the area of the throat where their thyroid is located but we still need to have more accurate and more objective information.

TSH and thyroid antibody lab results tell us how well a person is recovering and indicate when it's time to move from the Phase I to the Phase II protocol. Therefore a physician is required to order these two lab tests.

3. Evaluating other thyroid hormones.

Reducing thyroid antibodies and thyroid inflammation is the first step. The second step or Phase II is all about maximizing or optimizing thyroid hormone production.

There are 4 primary thyroid lab tests needed for this evaluation. These tests are TSH, Total T4, Free T4 and Free T3.

You already know the reasons for lowering and monitoring TSH. Yet when your thyroid antibodies are low enough and we enter Phase II of the program we want TSH to increase in order to stimulate your thyroid gland to make hormones again. We don't want to be dependent upon a thyroid medication if we can help it.

We monitor TSH in Phase I to be sure it is low enough. We monitor TSH in Phase II to be sure there's enough of the hormone to activate your thyroid cells to make thyroid hormones. If there is enough TSH stimulation we need to know how well the thyroid is responding.

The best test for evaluating how well the thyroid is responding is called Total T4. T4 is the primary thyroid hormone and "Total" includes both the T4 coupled or bound to its carrier protein as well as the T4 which is free and available.

Optimizing Total T4 levels requires two things. One is plenty of TSH stimulation, and the other is all the nutrients the thyroid needs to make its hormones. Missing just one of them leads to sub-optimal T4 thyroid hormone levels.

In Phase II, if a person's TSH is optimal but their Total T4 production is low then we know the problem is with the thyroid gland. Low Total T4 production is most often due to a lack of thyroid nutrients, yet in the case of Hashimoto's, this low production can be due to years of antibody activity and thyroid inflammation, and some degree of thyroid scaring and destruction.

Even though the lab test for Total T4 does provide us with important information we still need to know how much is free. If most of the T4 is bound and very little of it is free then a person will suffer from low thyroid hormones even though their thyroid is working well. When most of the T4 is bound the problem is not with the thyroid gland but a problem with excessive binding of T4 to proteins.

To evaluate how much of the Total T4 is free we use the Free T4 lab test. So if we have a normal Total T4 with a low Free T4 then we know that the person's T4 is mostly bound due to elevated estrogens, deficient progesterone or poor liver function.

And even when TSH is optimal and Total T4 is optimal and Free T4 is optimal a person can still suffer from low thyroid hormone symptoms. Why is this?

T4 is referred to as the mother or pro-hormone because it is used to make other thyroid hormones, the most important being T3 or triiodothyronine.   It is very important... I repeat it is <u>very important</u> for you to know that T4 is not the thyroid hormone that activates every cell in your body. The primary activating thyroid hormone is T3. This fact has been forgotten by many physicians.

This hormone, T3, is formed by removing one atom of iodine from T4. Miraculous don't you think? This single step of removing an atom of iodine can make the difference between a life of vitality and one of fatigue and apathy.

Fortunately there is a lab test for T3 known as Free T3. This helps us to evaluate how well a person is converting Free T4 to Free T3.

If Free T3 is low while all other thyroid lab tests are optimal then this is a conversion problem.

Lab testing is vital for understanding all the possible causes of low thyroid hormone symptoms and having a physician to order these tests is essential.

This is not a solo journey. You cannot do this with natural products alone. You must know when it's time to move through the different phases of resolving Hashimoto's and this requires lab testing.

SECTION 2

NINE CRUCIAL MISTAKES

"Mistakes are the usual bridge between inexperience and wisdom. "

Phyllis Therous

Believing Hashimoto's is a Disease

All of us want to know that our actions are leading us in the direction of our desired results. With Hashimoto's, what results are we hoping for? Can we believe that a <u>disease</u> such as Hashimoto's is curable? Let me word that question a little differently. Can we believe that a <u>condition</u> such as Hashimoto's is curable? The wording is subtle but very different.

As an example, let's say that a person has a cluster of symptoms; skin eruptions when exposed to sunlight, some hair loss, insomnia, diarrhea, some mental confusion, swelling of hands and feet, and their gait or walk seems a bit clumsy and awkward.

They consult their physician who does the standard battery of lab tests and finds nothing out of the ordinary. The person is told that everything is fine and not to worry, "It's probably just due to stress." Yet the person instinctively knows that something is wrong.

They visit another physician who prescribes a medication for the diarrhea and sleeping pills for the insomnia. Both help with the symptoms but still the person doesn't feel well.

A third physician recommends seeing a psychiatrist and we all know where that road leads.

Finally a fourth physician recognizes the pattern of symptoms and gives the diagnosis of Pellagra. At first the person is relieved. Finally someone understands them, but then there's the concern of having a disease.

After some reassurance the physician tells the person that this condition is caused by the lack of a B vitamin called niacin or B3. This is met with great relief. Administering niacin will clear the condition completely unless the nervous system has been damaged.

In some ways I believe that Hashimoto's is similar to Pellagra in that it is a condition arising from a variety of nutrient deficiencies. Whatever may be the cause of lowered thyroid hormone production (lack of iodide, zinc, selenium, etc.), it will result in the elevation of TSH, which is the first step leading to thyroid inflammation.

This initial increase in TSH even has a name or diagnosis. It's called Subclinical Hypothyroidism (SCH). It doesn't always develop into Hashimoto's but a high percentage of people with SCH do develop this Hashimoto's.

To recover from Hashimoto's requires lowering both TSH and thyroid antibodies while quenching the fire of thyroid inflammation and supplying specific nutrients for the thyroid gland.

Believing that Hashimoto's is an incurable disease is the first mistake people make.

Focusing on Visualization & Psychology

Picturing health and believing in the body's innate ability to heal is extremely important yet it's not enough. I know about the power of intention and the use of positive affirmations. It has its place.

Here is a brief quote from Robert Collier's book *The Secret of the Ages.*

"You fear ill health, when if you would concentrate that same amount of thought upon good health you would insure the very condition you fear to lose. Functional disturbances are caused solely by the mind through wrong thinking. The remedy for them is not a drug but right thinking, for the trouble is not in the organs but in the mind."

So much of this passage is true. And though it's important to tap into this inner source of healing, we <u>must</u> simultaneously recognize that if the cause of our condition is the lack of nutrients then no matter what, the body cannot repair itself and cannot regain its health even if we could walk on water.

In 1930 Dr. Weston Price published a book called *Nutrition and Physical Degeneration*. In previous decades to its publication Price had traveled around the world to remote and isolated regions examining the health of people eating only foods produced in their region. This was, of course, way before the time of pesticides, herbicides and the thousands of chemicals we are exposed to these days.

Over many years Price kept returning to each location to observe the health of succeeding generations. The only variable in his study was the importation of foods from other regions of the world. These imported foods had passed through various manufacturing processes, meaning they were altered from their original state and thus inferior in nutrient quality compared with what these people were used to. Through photographs and other documentation, Price recorded obvious physical signs of degenerative disease in these people who had once lived in perfect health.

I mention Dr. Price's book to emphasize that illness has the dual component of both psychology and nutrition and with Hashimoto's we must emphasize the nutritional side.

The second mistake people make is the belief that they can overcome their condition through the mind and heart without consideration of nutrient rich foods.

Relying Only on a Thyroid Prescription

It's becoming more and more obvious that the medical system is flawed when it comes to <u>curing</u> chronic ailments. People often become irritated when speaking about their personal experiences with their physician, especially those with Hashimoto's. They are generally fed up with not getting the answers or the help they need.

Think about it. What logical sense does it make to only be offered a thyroid hormone prescription for a thyroid autoimmune disease?

We know that a thyroid prescription will lower TSH and we now understand why this is important. Doctors also know that the prescription will lower TSH however I'm not sure if they understand why lowering TSH is helpful for Hashimoto's.

Thinking that a thyroid prescription is all that's needed is faulty thinking because it does nothing to lower inflammation (except by lowering TSH and thus H2O2) nor does it help to repair any damage to the thyroid. The prescription also does not address the thyroid's need to be nourished in order to improve its function and production of its hormones.

It's important for you to understand what the typical thyroid hormone prescription actually is.

Since the late 1800's physicians prescribed animal thyroid gland to people with hypothyroidism. These preparations contained the same thyroid hormones (T4, T3 and others) found in our own thyroid gland.

This approach worked very well, yet as you may know Big Pharma can only produce pharmaceuticals that can be patented and you cannot patent something that's naturally occurring such as a hormone. So the chemical structure of our own thyroid hormone (T4) was modified slightly in order to patent it.

In 1958 the first synthetic thyroid hormone came on the market and was called Synthroid (_syn_thetic _**thyroid**_). The marketing pitch to doctors was that the concentration or milligram dosage of the synthetic was more accurate and consistent than animal or pig thyroid. In the 60's there was a huge propaganda campaign that hit many popular women's magazines which focused on the symptoms of hypothyroidism. This was one of the first campaigns that sent the public into their physician's office asking for a medication. Today this style of marketing is everywhere.

The problem is that Synthroid and all similar thyroid pharmaceuticals such as levoxyl and levothyroxine contain only the T4 thyroid hormone. But T4 is not the activating thyroid hormone. T3 is.

You can have all the T4 in the world floating through your veins but if it isn't converted to T3 you will suffer from low thyroid hormone symptoms.

The reason why so many people with Hashimoto's feel better, when initially taking the synthetic thyroid hormone, is because it lowers TSH that in turn lowers inflammation. Yet this improvement is only partial because Hashimoto's patients are unable to optimally convert the T4 into T3.

There are several options to improve T3 levels that will be covered in another section.

The third mistake people make is thinking that all they need to treat Hashimoto's is a thyroid prescription.

Thinking There's No Harm in Taking a Thyroid Medication

Each time someone reaches for that little amber prescription bottle they experience a subtle message that they are not well, that something is wrong with them, that something within them is not working correctly. It also develops a sense of dependency not only upon the medication but upon their physician and the medical system.

This sense of being ill and dependent must be removed from the psyche if a person is to become well. I'll make a very bold statement here to make a point even though I know it has exceptions. Hashimoto's, Primary Hypothyroidism and Secondary Hypothyroidism all have the same origin.

Here are the three related conditions;

~ Hashimoto's

~ Primary Hypothyroidism with increased TSH and low thyroid hormone production

~ Secondary Hypothyroidism with low TSH and low thyroid hormone production

Generally speaking all 3 originate from the same cause, that being deficiencies of essential nutrients. Yes, there are your thyroid cysts and growths as well as inhibiting environmental substances but for the majority of people these three relate to nutrient deficiencies.

Thyroid medication is often necessary to help a person feel better yet it does nothing to address the lack of nutrients which is the source of their problem. These nutrients include iodine, iodide, zinc, selenium, iron, essential fatty acids and others.

Hashimoto's, Primary, and Secondary Hypothyroidism should be a flashing light, a signal alerting people and their physicians that something is fundamentally out of balance. Being handed a prescription does nothing to explain the reasons for their condition, nor does taking a pill motivate people to change.

As far as I know no one has ever died from Hashimoto's or Hypothyroidism yet other more severe conditions can result from them. Take breast disease and breast cancer as only two examples of what may result when Hashimoto's and hypothyroidism remain untreated from several fronts.

One study out of Italy took a group of women recently diagnosed with ductal cell breast cancer and checked them for thyroid issues. Forty-six percent of them had a thyroid problem. The majority of these had either a thyroid goiter (enlarged) most often due to an iodide deficiency, or they had Hashimoto's.

Taking a thyroid prescription can be harmful because it doesn't address the underlying deficiencies and the body's need for these health promoting nutrients, continuing to leave the person in a state of deficiency and susceptibility.

The fourth mistake people make is thinking that a thyroid prescription is resolving their autoimmune condition.

Believing Iodine is Good for Their Thyroid

This subject is extremely important because high dose iodine and potassium iodide can cause some acute and chronic problems that can be avoided through lab test screening and a more conservative approach.

I have seen a number of people in relatively good health shift into a hyperthyroid condition due to high dosing of iodine and iodide. Do not fool around with high doses of iodide and iodine UNLESS your thyroid antibodies are normal and even then start by administering it very slowly.

With one woman we first checked her thyroid antibodies before starting iodine and iodide and they were normal. After 4 months of taking high doses she developed Hashimoto's along with hyperthyroid symptoms. From my perspective, this present wave of taking high doses is dangerous. Everyone, before taking high doses, needs to be checked for antibodies AND to improve their selenium and glutathione levels. I'll soon explain why this is important.

A 68 year old woman with a slightly high TSH of 4.3 and low Total T4 was prescribed 25 mg of the combination iodine and potassium iodide. Providing some iodide is often all the thyroid needs to boost its production of thyroid hormones.

After 4 months we rechecked her TSH. It had shot up to 107!!! Her M.D. in Vancouver freaked, which sent her running to me.

I knew her elevated TSH was a response to the iodine and iodide so I gave her plenty of reassurance along with the reasons why the body increases its production of TSH. Within a month of being off the product her TSH was back to normal and she's still doing really well.

Just imagine what might have happened if she had Hashimoto's. For this reason I check everyone for thyroid antibodies before recommending higher doses of iodine and iodide.

Another case was a young man in good health. He had been experimenting with higher doses of the same product, taking between 50 and 100mg daily. He developed two thyroid cysts and experienced all the symptoms of hyperthyroidism including a resting heart rate of 110 beats per minute, weight loss, intolerance of exercise and a voracious appetite.

Even after two months after discontinuing the iodine and iodide product his symptoms remained. The advice from three physicians was to radiate his thyroid.

Fortunately we started him on high doses of vitamin C along with the removal of his single dental filling and some heavy metal chelation. His symptoms improved within two weeks and his thyroid hormones returned to normal after another month. He is very well now but will never touch an iodine and iodide product again.

There's another concern I have regarding high doses of iodide. You'll find in every current medical physiology text a phenomenon called the 'Wolff-Chaikoff' effect. The proponents of high dosing of iodide and iodine say this effect does not exist.

The effect goes something like this. When "the intake of iodide exceeds 2mg per day the intraglandular concentration of iodide reaches a level that inhibits the iodide trap" as well as the synthesis or production of thyroid hormones.

These traps are mentioned later on. They are also called Sodium Iodide Symports, specialized channels on the membranes of thyroid cells which absorb iodide. When these are inhibited, less iodide is absorbed and thyroid hormone production declines. I have found this to be true.

Here are more results on the lady I just mentioned whom we recommended 25 mg of the combination of iodide and iodine. As you can see her TSH was a little on the high side (optimal being 2.0). Again, I felt it was high because her T4 was suboptimal, so the pituitary was producing more TSH trying to stimulate her thyroid to make more T4. I felt that giving her some iodide would provide more of this essential nutrient which thyroid cells require to increase their production.

LabCorp

LabCorp Seattle
550 17th Avenue, Ste 300
Seattle, WA 98122-5789

Phone: 206-861-7000

Specimen Number	Patient ID	Control Number	Account Number	Account Phone Number	Route
226-129-0471-0	90567	62015013168	09149190	954-922-1257	09

Thyroid Panel with TSH

TSH	3.563	uIU/ml	0.350 – 5.50
Thyroxine (T4)	6.1	ug/dL	4.5 – 12.0
Triiodothyronine, Free	3.6	pg/mL	2.3 – 4.2

The Triiodothyronine is the Free T3.

After six months we repeated her labs to find out the effects of the iodide and iodine.

Below you'll see that her TSH went from 3.563 to 107.49. Incredible!

And the Wolff-Chaikoff effect also showed up. Even though the TSH was outrageously high her thyroid's production of T4 dropped as well as her Free T3.

LabCorp	LabCorp Seattle 550 17th Avenue Ste 300 Seattle, WA 98122			Phone: 206-861-7000	
Specimen Number 072-129-2311-0	Patient ID	Control Number 53910198788	Account Number 09149190	Account Phone Number 954-922-1257	Route 09

TSH	107.490	**High**	uIU/ml	0.350 – 5.50
Thyroxine (T4), Free	0.46	**Low**	ng/dL	0.61 – 1.76
Triiodothyronine, Free	2.2	**Low**	pg/mL	2.3 – 4.2

I am, to say the least, extremely cautious with using high doses of iodine and iodide. My greatest concern for anyone using these trace minerals is if they have a thyroid autoimmune condition. With the study I mentioned earlier, where half of the people having no personal or family history of thyroid problems showed elevated TPO antibodies, I am concerned with the indiscriminate use of iodine and iodide.

First, do not harm!!

I believe that for someone whose thyroid antibodies are normal, a safe dose is a 3mg combination of iodine (1.25mg) and potassium iodide (1.75mg) in combination with 200-400mcg of selenium methionine. Research confirms the effectiveness of 3mg for cystic breast disease without any abnormal side effects.

Some people may need to be on higher doses than 3mg but they should be followed by a physician to be certain that their antibodies are not increasing.

For now, in this first phase of treatment and until your antibodies are within the normal range, you will need to avoid iodine and iodide. This means all sources found in supplements and specific foods.

The fifth mistake people make is thinking iodine and iodide are helpful for treating Hashimoto's.

The Avoidance of Iodine is for Life

The advice to stay away from iodide and iodine often comes from a physician who believes that these are the cause of Hashimoto's. Yet there are other physicians who say it doesn't really matter if you take them as long as it's not too much, yet they are vague about what is meant by "too much." Others say you need it, selling products for Hashimoto's that include kelp which is rich in iodine and iodide.

No wonder so many people are confused about treating Hashimoto's.

Yes, your physician is right to recommend restricting iodine and iodide but at the same time you cannot live a healthy life without it. Once your thyroid antibodies are down, these trace minerals must be slowly reintroduced. Eventually you need to saturate your tissues with iodine, especially breast, ovarian and prostate tissues.

The body has an innate ability to recognize that certain nutrients are essential for its survival and has thus developed the means of storing these nutrients.

Iron is stored as ferritin, a kind of iron protein carrier circulating in the blood. Vitamin B12 is stored in the liver for up to 5 years. In some ways the activating thyroid hormone T3 is stored as T4 which acts as a kind of reservoir or buffer. Iodine is stored in various tissues and provides added protection from environmental toxins and infections.

Through eons of generations the body figured out that the availability of iodine and iodide was variable depending upon season, harvest, and our migration, and it determined a means of storing them for those times of scarcity.

For iodide and iodine to be absorbed into various tissues they must pass through specific channels called NIS or Sodium Iodide Symports. To increase the number of these channels and to upregulate (stimulate) them to absorb iodine and iodide, the hormone TSH is required. So when we eat iodine rich foods or ingest iodine and iodide supplements, the body increases TSH production to help with their absorption.[18] [19] [20] [21]

The sixth mistake people make is thinking iodine and iodide must be avoided for the rest of their lives.

Using the Natural Approach by Avoiding a Thyroid Prescription

Many of us will try anything to avoid taking a prescription. It may be our intuition which steers us away thinking that drugs don't really cure, don't address the cause, and that they all have side effects.

I'm sure you have visited the home of a friend or family member and have sneaked a peak in what's called the medicine cabinet, to find it chock full of prescription bottles. Help me!

Many of us have educated ourselves about nutrition and have experienced the overall benefits of including more nutrient rich foods. It only makes sense that if we provide the body with what it needs, we can then maintain or recover our health.

Yet Hashimoto's is slightly different from some of the common conditions that respond well to nutritional and lifestyle changes.

There was a woman in her late 50's who had tried everything to treat her thyroid and for several years had avoided gluten, taken loads of supplements, and tried homeopathy and acupuncture.

As a side note, I do believe in acupuncture and I've practiced homeopathy for 30 years, however neither of these can ever be the singular approach since most thyroid issues including Hashimoto's result from nutrient deficiencies.

This woman had been diagnosed by her M.D. as being hypothyroid and he insisted on her taking a thyroid prescription which she refused. At her first consult we reviewed her lab results from over the years. They showed fluctuating TSH levels, so we decided to check her thyroid antibodies.

She had Hashimoto's. Within 3 weeks of starting her program that included a thyroid prescription and the avoidance of iodine and iodide, many of her symptoms improved, some dramatically.

She was the typical case of someone who wanted to do it naturally because her mindset was opposed to taking a pharmaceutical.

I need to add some clarity here about prescriptions. Generally the action of over-the-counter and prescription drugs is to oppose the body's symptoms. Taking aspirin or Tylenol will oppose the body's innate ability to produce a fever. This category of medicines is called "antipyretics" (against the fire).

For inflammation we use anti-inflammatory drugs. For depression we use anti-depressants. For pain we use analgesics. For hypertension we use an anti-hypertensive.

Prescriptions are designed to oppose. They are easy to take and give immediate relief. They are the Jack-in-the-Box or Doc-in-the-Box approach.

Many of us recognize that our symptoms are often tied to stress, to the lack of exercise, to not eating properly, and to not being able to relax. We decide to address the reasons for our physical and emotional symptoms rather than turning to a drug or chemical that will oppose or suppress them.

When thyroid hormone production first begins to slip our bodies produce a variety of subtle symptoms. These could be slight constipation, a little weight gain that we can't seem to lose, some thinning of the hair, feeling on the chilly side, dryer skin, and many others. Over years and decades these symptoms become worse until finally our thyroid is investigated. If it's low enough we are given a thyroid prescription.

But what does this mean that we now need a thyroid prescription? This prescription simply adds additional thyroid hormones onto the small amount our thyroid is producing. Obviously a thyroid medication does not oppose symptoms. It simply helps to optimize thyroid hormone levels in the blood stream.

The attitude people have about being natural is <u>very</u> important. This mindset fits the wellness part of the Hashimoto's program BUT most people will need a thyroid hormone prescription at the beginning of the first phase of treatment.

The seventh mistake people make is to believe that they can recover from Hashimoto's without a thyroid prescription.

Trusting their Doctors to Order the Right Lab Tests

Interpreting thyroid lab tests is a huge subject that I'll explain a little later on in another section. But here's an example of why your doctor may not know which labs are most important.

To determine if a person's symptoms are actually due to low thyroid hormones, if you had to choose just _one_ test, which would it be? Which thyroid hormone is the most important one to check?

Certainly you want to know to what extent the thyroid is being stimulated so TSH is important.

You also want to know how well the thyroid is able to respond to TSH, so it's essential to check the level of the primary thyroid hormone, T4.

But which thyroid hormone stimulates the metabolism of almost every cell in the body? Which one is essential for the production of energy? It's T3 and you need to know how much of this T3 is free to travel outside the blood stream and enter the membranes of cells to trigger metabolism.

So the winner is….T3!!!

Yes, all the thyroid hormone blood tests are very important, but testing for Free T3 levels is the most important when investigating low thyroid hormone symptoms.

But I'd venture to say that maybe only 5% of physicians check T3. Most check for only TSH and Free T4.

One more note just for clarification. With Hashimoto's we are only concerned with two lab tests in the beginning. These are TSH and the thyroid antibodies. This is all we care about. With Hashimoto's the levels of T4 and T3 fluctuate so much that they cannot be used for any practical purpose.

Doctors usually dose a thyroid prescription based on lab results and the size of the person.

However this will often not work with Hashimoto's and can even backfire. Prescribing a thyroid medication in order to lower TSH must be solely based upon the person's symptoms. I know this can be like driving a car at night without the headlights on but this is how doctors practiced "thyroidology" for over 60 years, before we had thyroid lab tests. Using a person's symptoms for adjusting a thyroid prescription is not quackery but an essential first step in Phase I of treating Hashimoto's.

If any doctor believes they can prescribe a thyroid medication based upon the lab results of a person with Hashimoto's then they don't understand the hormone level fluctuations that almost all Hashimoto's patients experience.

The eighth mistake people make is relying on a physician who doesn't understand the full spectrum of thyroid lab tests and how to prescribe for Hashimoto's as compared with a hypothyroid patient.

Starting with the Conventional Dose of Thyroid Medication

A conventional dose of thyroid medication is typically given to someone when the diagnosis is Hypothyroidism. This is not how you want to start if you have Hashimoto's because this will often cause an intensification of symptoms. The hypo days may be better, yet often the hyper days get pretty crazy. It's important to prescribe thyroid medication in a specific way to avoid an aggravation.

It's important to know that Hashimoto's is considered to be the primary cause of Hypothyroidism so let's first look at the two 2 types of hypothyroidism and how they are differentiated through lab testing. One is called Primary Hypothyroidism and the other is called Secondary Hypothyroidism.

Here are the similarities between the two:

~   They both have low thyroid hormone production.

~   Their symptoms can be identical.

~ They have both experienced decades of low thyroid hormones until reaching the final stage of requiring a prescription.

~ They can both be treated with the same thyroid prescription.

What are the differences between Primary and Secondary?

~ Primary has high TSH with *low thyroid hormone production.*

~ Secondary has low TSH with *low thyroid hormone production.*

Primary's reason for low thyroid hormone production is because, even though the thyroid is getting plenty of TSH stimulation, it lacks the nutrients it needs to make its hormones. You are beginning to understand that the primary reason for developing Hashimoto's is also for the same reason, thyroid cells not getting the nutrients they need to make their hormones.

Secondary's reason for low thyroid hormone production is because the pituitary is not producing enough TSH to stimulate the thyroid to make its hormones. Low TSH results in low thyroid hormone production.

It's so simple, yes?

So how are Primary and Secondary different from Hashimoto's when it comes to the prescription of a thyroid medication?

This is extremely important to understand because if a person with Hashimoto's is prescribed a thyroid medication in the same way it's prescribed for Primary Hypothyroidism then their recovery from Hashimoto's may be delayed.

From now on when I use the term hypothyroidism I am referring to Primary Hypothyroidism.

Hypothyroidism, when unrelated to Hashimoto's, comes on very slowly over years and decades. It is a <u>steady</u> decline in the production of thyroid hormones without huge fluctuations in either TSH or thyroid hormone levels. TSH slowly increases as thyroid hormone production slowly declines.

The scenario is quite different from Hashimoto's with its thyroid cell destruction and the sudden release of thyroid hormones.

When thyroid hormones are prescribed for hypothyroidism the initial dose is often very close to the dose they'll be taking for the rest of their lives.

The T4 in the thyroid prescription is almost identical to the T4 made by the person's thyroid gland. Both the synthetic T4 and the

T4 produced by their thyroid last for quite a while before they are broken down and excreted. Half the time it takes the body to fully metabolize or break down either the T4 in the drug or the T4 made by the thyroid gland is referred to as its half-life. T4's half-life is about seven days.

In practice this means that about half of the T4 that's swallowed on day one will still be in the blood stream on the 7th day. So when a person is taking their thyroid medication every day during that first week, the T4 in the blood will slowly climb until it reaches a plateau, a steady state. At this point there is very little fluctuation in levels of T4 even if a person misses a dose.

During week one, as T4 rises, TSH, as a result, will begin to decline. And as TSH declines, the person's thyroid hormone production also declines.

I hope you can see why people often feel better in those first few weeks of beginning a thyroid medication. They initially have a lot more circulating T4 because they've added T4 to their already existing T4. Yet over time, as their TSH level declines, their own thyroid hormone production also declines.

At some point a person put on thyroid medication will return to their physician for an evaluation and a follow up blood test. Most doctors check only TSH to be sure it's down. Most of the time the thyroid dose will be adjusted according to TSH results rather than the patient's symptoms.

So why can't we prescribe a thyroid medication in the same way for Hashimoto's?

Hashimoto's is an autoimmune condition involving white blood cells, thyroid inflammation, and the destruction of thyroid cells. With Hashimoto's, thyroid hormones in the blood stream are constantly fluctuating because some thyroid cells will break apart, leaking thyroid hormones. This is very different from the steady thyroid hormone state of hypothyroidism.

If you prescribe thyroid hormones for a Hashimoto's patient in the same way as you would for hypothyroidism you will create greater peaks in thyroid hormones. These thyroid hormone peaks are the combination of the hormones leaking for broken thyroid cells, the thyroid prescription and those being made by the thyroid.

Not only will this create hyperthyroid symptoms but it's very possible that the body will begin to protect itself from elevated thyroid hormones by making another thyroid hormone called Reverse T3. This thyroid hormone, made from T4, will block the activating thyroid hormone T3, kind of like putting on the brakes of a speeding car.

Remember, every hormone has a half-life. While T4's half-life is seven days, the half-life of TSH is only about one hour.[22] Its production is fairly steady when thyroid hormone production is also steady. But Hashimoto's can have these outbursts of T4. As thyroid hormones fluctuate so will TSH, and this is why when reviewing a series of TSH lab tests you'll see great variations in TSH levels.

It's like the person driving through a hilly area, who is constantly pressing and releasing the gas pedal, press, release, press, release, just to continue up and down the hills at the same speed. These are the ups and downs of TSH levels.

So prescribing thyroid medication for Hashimoto's in the same way as you would for hypothyroidism just doesn't work very well.

Remember, the first goal of treating Hashimoto's is to reduce TSH without creating a situation of having too much T4. For this reason the initial dose of thyroid medication must be very low, about one-third to one-fourth of what the normal dose would be for hypothyroidism. The desired effect of prescribing in this way is to help steady the production of TSH as it slowly declines. This decline in TSH will slow the thyroid's production of thyroid hormones along with a decline in hydrogen peroxide production and thyroid inflammation. Every 7-10 days, after evaluating the person's symptoms, the thyroid prescription is again increased by another small increment.

The ninth mistake people make is approaching the pharmaceutical treatment of Hashimoto's as if it were hypothyroidism.

SECTION 3

DEDICATE 3 MONTHS TO

RECOVERING YOUR HEALTH

"My great hope is to laugh as much as I cry; to get my work done and try to love somebody and have the courage to accept the love in return."

Maya Angelou

Phase I

The first phase is the most important and will require the greatest effort and determination on your part. It requires becoming educated, thinking in new and unfamiliar ways, altering some personal habits, and taking initiative.

On the physical or biochemical level the primary goals of this first phase are the following:

~ Lowering TSH to 1.0 or less

~ Decreasing thyroid inflammation

~ Priming the thyroid with all the essential nutrients it needs, excluding iodine & iodide

~ Repairing thyroid damage

Reduce Thyroid Inflammation by Lowering TSH

First I'll categorize the three primary clinical situations in which most people find themselves.

Group 1- These individuals have tried to treat their Hashimoto's naturally without taking a thyroid prescription. Some are taking a thyroid glandular supplement thinking this will help. But most thyroid glandulars do not have any active thyroid hormone in them and even the few that do contain only the single thyroid hormone T3. This T3 may help them to feel more energetic yet it is not enough to lower TSH. Both T4 and T3 are necessary to decrease TSH.

Group 2- Individuals in this group are already taking a thyroid prescription. Maybe they were first diagnosed with Primary Hypothyroidism and later on Hashimoto's was discovered, or they were diagnosed with Hashimoto's from the very beginning.

Group 3- These individuals are also taking a thyroid prescription. When they were diagnosed their TSH was low. They could have first been diagnosed with Secondary Hypothyroidism and later with Hashimoto's or simply diagnosed with Hashimoto's from the very beginning.

If you are not sure whether you are in Group 2 or 3 it doesn't matter too much when it comes to treatment.

If you are in **Group 1** your antibodies are most often elevated because your TSH is high. The only way I know of to lower your TSH is by increasing thyroid hormone levels and the only way I've discovered to do this is through the use of a thyroid medication.

If you are in **Group 2** you must be sure you are taking enough thyroid medication to get your TSH below 1.0. If your TSH is less than 1.0 then there is no need to increase your dose. Reducing your antibodies is simply a matter of cooling down the thyroid with antioxidants, repairing your thyroid and altering your diet. Your recovery in Phase II will likely be fairly rapid. If you are taking the synthetic thyroid medication of T4 you should consider either adding T3 to it or getting a compounded T4 and T3 prescription.

Your conversion of T4 to T3 is likely less than optimal and adding T3 would improve your metabolism and increase your energy, helping you to recover more quickly.

If you are in **Group 3** you must also be sure that you are taking enough thyroid prescription to lower your TSH to below 1.0. Your recovery in Phase II will probably take longer because you may have had Hashimoto's longer. You should also consider modifying your prescription as mentioned in the previous section for **Group 2**.

Now let's talk about thyroid prescriptions.

Selecting the Best Thyroid Prescription

There are basically 4 types of thyroid medications to choose from.

The first type is the one prescribed by most M.D.'s which is Synthroid, L-thyroxin or Levothyroxine. These medications are synthetic and mimic the T4 or thyroxin which the thyroid makes. T4, whether it's from our thyroid or the synthetic, is the primary thyroid hormone that regulates the level of TSH. When T4 goes up then TSH comes down.

T4 is not the primary thyroid hormone that increases the activity of our cells. T4 must be changed into the activating T3 thyroid hormone. Many people don't convert T4 into T3 all that well and will often experience only moderate improvement when taking the synthetic T4 thyroid medication. This is the disadvantage of taking Synthroid or L-thyroxin, that it contains only T4 and not T3.

The second prescription medication is called Cytomel or T3. This is often added to the synthetic Synthroid or L-thyroxin. Some people prefer not switching from their synthetic T4 medication for a number of reasons including their insurance coverage. Cytomel is simply added to their T4 prescription and thus provides the activating thyroid hormone.

The third thyroid prescription medication is made from the thyroid gland of a pig. This has been used by physicians for many decades with the current ones being Armour Thyroid and Naturthroid. There are others as well. We've tried thyroid glands from other animals but pig works best, just as we used to use the insulin from pig pancreas for years.

Pig thyroid cells contain both hormones T4 and T3 in the same ratio as our own thyroid cells. This medication helps to lower TSH and provides T3 to help those who don't convert T4 to T3 well.

I have used this form of thyroid medication for Hashimoto's but have stopped. The reason is because when this glandular is swallowed and the pig thyroid cells are broken apart by the enzymes in the stomach, both the enzyme thyroperoxidase and the protein thyroglobulin are released. If and when this enzyme and protein are absorbed through the small intestine, the immune system will be triggered since with Hashimoto's the antibodies are primed and on the lookout for either one of these or both. Using the desiccated thyroid glandular will, in many cases, perpetuate thyroid antibody activity.

I have switched instead to the use of the compounded T4 and T3 for this reason although I still prescribe the glandular for other thyroid problems.

The last type of thyroid prescription is a combination of T4 and T3 which are both synthetic and compounded by special pharmacies. This form can be adjusted to whatever micrograms the physician asks for. This is the form I prefer for treating Hashimoto's.

Various ingredients in addition to the thyroid hormones are added to these capsules. The prevalent preparation by almost all compounding pharmacies is the slow release form. It took me awhile to figure out that this preparation just wasn't working for a lot of patients.

Those who first consulted me, who were taking Armour and who weren't feeling all that bad even though their antibodies were elevated, found that when we switched to the equivalent dose of the compounded, slow release T4 and T3 they didn't feel all that well.

We tested their TSH levels when they were on the Armour and then repeated the test when they'd been on the compounded after one month. One lady's TSH went from around 1.0 on Armour to 3.8 on the compounded.

What this means is that the amount of circulating thyroid hormones from the compounded was less, thus the TSH rose. Since she was on an equivalent dose of the T4 and T3 this meant that she wasn't absorbing it, that the ingredient used to slow down the absorption of T4 and T3 was actually preventing the hormones from being completely absorbed.

Therefore I recommend only the immediate release and prefer the rice filler and the vege caps as well.

If a person has obvious candida symptoms with a white or gray coated tongue then I know that their small intestine's ability to absorb medication is compromised. In this case I have the compounding pharmacy mix the T4 and T3 in a cocoa butter lozenge to be dissolved under the tongue. Most of it will enter the blood circulation and if any is swallowed at least it will not be bound to some kind cellulose.

Prescribing Incremental Doses for Hashimoto's

How a thyroid medication is prescribed is very important for a number of reasons. As a reminder, you cannot prescribe a thyroid medication for a person with Hashimoto's based upon thyroid lab results because TSH and thyroid hormone levels are constantly fluctuating.

The first goal of prescribing is to stabilize and lower TSH. When thyroid hormones go up in the blood TSH comes down, yet if we prescribe too high of a dose with Hashimoto's then the combination of the thyroid prescription and the release of thyroid hormones due to thyroid cell inflammation and destruction, can easily cause hyper symptoms often resulting in excess of T4 and sometimes elevated Reverse T3.

The way to prescribe thyroid hormones for Hashimoto's is to begin with very low doses, about one-third or one-fourth of what is normally prescribed for hypothyroidism. Because of T4's long half-life (seven days), this daily third or quarter dose will slowly increase T4 levels in the blood.

The change in levels of T3, when taking a compounded T4 and T3, is different because the half-life of T3 is around 8-12 hours. Thus when taking Cytomel or a compounded T4 and T3, a person immediately experiences the benefits of T3 as it rises and falls after each dose. Because of this short half-life and the rise and fall in blood concentrations, T3 and compounded T4 & T3 must be taken twice daily, about 8-10 hours part.

It is common to feel an immediate improvement during the first 4-7 days of taking any of the thyroid medications. Around the fifth day a person often experiences a slight step backwards in their energy. There's a sense that the medication is not working, but this is not true.

The reason for this step backwards is because when the thyroid prescription first enters the blood stream on day one, the T4 is added to the thyroid hormones being produced by their own thyroid. The person now has more circulating T4 plus the T3 it is converting into. Since T4 lasts for such a long time before it is broken down or metabolized, each day more and more T4 is being added to the circulation. This feels good.

But as the T4 from the medication increases circulating levels each day, TSH levels begin to decline. This decline lowers thyroid stimulation and thus lowers your thyroid's production of its hormones. But remember that T4 has a half life of 7 days so the experience of this decline of thyroid hormone production due to decreasing TSH levels won't be felt for about 7 days.

Thus levels of T4 and T3 in the blood will initially increase and then, in about a week, they will slightly decline since thyroid hormone production is less. This experience of feeling better followed by a mild sense of relapse happens each time a person with Hashimoto's increases their thyroid medication.

So if a person feels only somewhat better after the first 10 to 14 days of taking the first third or quarter dose, they will need to increase it again by another third or quarter dose. For many people, this second increase may be enough. They'll feel better and sense they don't need to increase by another dose.

Those individuals needing more should continue to increase their thyroid dose every 10 days until they reach a state of feeling really well. For some this could go on until they've reached the equivalent of 2 grains over approximately 2 months.

Most people will instinctively know when they've arrived at the right dose. Anyone going a little over their optimal dose will experience a more rapid heart rate and feel a little hyper. Adjusting down by a third or quarter dose will bring them back to a state of feeling well and more balanced.

If you are in **Group 2** or **3** and are already taking a synthetic T4 medication with a TSH above 1.0, then I suggest adding Cytomel or switching to the compounded T4 and T3.

I think you understand the reason for adding the T3 by now.

T3 or Cytomel comes in a variety of strengths. I suggest starting at 5mcg twice daily about 10 hours apart. Do this for about 3-5 days before going any higher. Do not be in a hurry. You can then try splitting the 12.5mcg tablet taking a half tablet again twice daily for another week before going up from there.

Once you've found your preferred dose of thyroid medication and are feeling well, have your TSH levels checked after about 2 weeks. If it is still greater than 1.0 you'll need to increase your thyroid hormone prescription by another third or quarter of what you are taking.

Therefore if you are on 100mcg of Synthroid or Levothyroxine you will add 25 to 35mcg.

These are simple guidelines to allow you to have an open discussion with your physician. You will, from what I've told you, have a sense of whether your physician knows what they are talking about. If they don't, thank them and move on to find a physician who does.

If you find your physician to be uncooperative or can't find one who is knowledgeable, we do offer long-distance consultations.

Now you know about the use of various thyroid prescriptions and their usefulness in lowering TSH. Next is another means of reducing TSH.

Eliminate Iodine & Iodide

For iodide to be absorbed into a thyroid cell it must be collected in what's called an iodide trap. The activity of this trap, and thus the absorption of iodide, is stimulated by TSH.[23]

When there's a deficiency of iodide, TSH will initially increase in order to capture as much iodide as possible for the thyroid. This increase in TSH, with somewhat normal thyroid hormones, is known as Subclinical Hypothyroidism (SCH). People with SCH, because of the elevated TSH, have a greater risk of developing Hashimoto's.

TSH also stimulates similar traps or channels in other cells and tissues, and when iodine and iodide are more available, TSH levels will increase to promote the absorption of iodide and iodine into these tissues.

A 2008 study in *Endocrinology Journal* demonstrated an increase in TSH levels in Japanese adults ingesting 15 and 30 grams of a seaweed called Kombu.[24] From this Japanese study as well as others we know that iodine and iodide increase TSH production for a very good reason, to increase the absorption of these trace minerals. Yet this is something we want to avoid with Hashimoto's.

Therefore, both the long term lack of, as well as the increased availability of iodine and iodide will increase TSH. For this reason, since we want to decrease TSH, it is important to pass through the Phase I of treating Hashimoto's as quickly as possible.

This is another reason for being on a thyroid hormone prescription because even though an iodide deficiency can eventually cause increased TSH, having plenty of circulating thyroid hormones will keep TSH down.

Besides being on an optimal dose of thyroid hormones, the approach to reducing TSH is the following;

~ Avoid iodine & iodide in supplements. Douglas Labs makes a multivitamin, UltraGenic, which does not contain iodine. Read labels.

~ Avoid foods high in iodine such as kelp, seaweed, shellfish and haddock. Other fish should be limited to 1-2 times per week. Fresh water fish are fine.

~ Avoid iodized (iodide) salt.

~ Sea salt can be used to taste.

~ Avoid kelp in supplements. This ingredient is often found in thyroid supplements.

Remember that the avoidance of iodine and iodide is temporary and as soon as TSH and thyroid antibodies are down we'll begin to reintroduce these two important elements immediately.

Nourish the Thyroid in Preparation for Phase II

By avoiding iodide it is next to impossible for the thyroid to make its hormones especially since TSH is being reduced.

Yet our eventual goal is to maximize the thyroid's production of thyroid hormones. This will take place in Phase II. In the meantime we need to prepare the thyroid by giving it the nutrients it will eventually need to make its hormones. We are, in a way, priming the thyroid so that when we reintroduce iodide in Phase II, thyroid cells will be ready to begin production.

Here are the nutrients that nourish the thyroid.

~ Selenium methionine, 400mcg taken once daily.

~ Zinc picolinate, 25-50mg taken once daily. The higher dose of 50mg is for anyone with the following; recurring colds or infections, rough skin, chest deformities (pectus excavatum), white spots on the finger nails, acne, celiac disease, stretch marks and poor wound healing.

~ Iron, but only if body iron stores are low or there's an iron deficiency anemia. Iron stores are best determined by the ferritin lab test and if levels are low the best product is Ferritin from Cardiovascular Research.

~ Vitamin A in the emulsified form is easiest to absorb. Biotics Research makes Bio-Ae-Mulsion Forte with one drop equaling 12,500 IU's. Taking 3 drops a day is recommended. This form can be taken for longer periods without affecting the liver. A pregnant woman should not take more than 10,000 IU's daily so one drop every other day is best.

~ Essential Fatty Acids, preferably with fish, flax and borage seed oils. Biotics makes Optimal EFA's which contains these.

~ Both B2 (riboflavin) and B3 as inositol hexanicotinate, 100mg and 500mg respectively. This is found in a product called ATP Cofactors by Optimox.

So we are reducing TSH through the use of a thyroid medication and the avoidance of iodine and iodide, and now we are priming the thyroid with nutrients. Next we need to reduce thyroid inflammation through the use of antioxidants.

Extinguish the Flame of Thyroid Inflammation

The labeling of Hashimoto's includes the term thyroiditis with "itis" referring to inflammation. Most people do not experience any sensation of inflammation in the area of their thyroid, while some do experience swelling, warmth, or discomfort.

This inflammation is due to the thyroid cell's production of hydrogen peroxide along with the activity of white blood cells in and around the thyroid. These white cells were originally attracted to the area when thyroid cells began to break apart leaking cell debris and hydrogen peroxide. Their initial role was to clean up the mess.

Selenium, because it's been proven to protect thyroid cells from destruction, plays a very important role in thyroid inflammation.[25]
[26] [27] [28]

With Hashimoto's, even when a person's TSH is low, the thyroid can still be caught in a vicious cycle of inflammation with increased white cell activity. It's sort of like a forest fire that's burning out of control. Antioxidants provide the means of cooling the thyroid and interrupting this destructive process. Once again selenium will interrupt this cycle by neutralizing excess hydrogen peroxide.[29]

The primary antioxidant studied in Hashimoto's medical research is glutathione. Glutathione has demonstrated very positive results in reducing thyroid antibodies.[30] [31] [32] [33] The primary means of improving circulating glutathione is by providing those nutrients the body needs to make its own glutathione.

Once again we come to the trace mineral, selenium, which is the premier nutrient for improving glutathione levels. A selenium deficiency has been associated with thyroid autoimmune disease [34] [35] [36] and many studies have shown how selenium is also important for reducing thyroid antibodies.[37] [38]

To illustrate how important selenium is in the treatment of AITD, one observational case from a medical journal published in December of 2008 studied a woman being treated for Hashimoto's. She had already been taking the thyroid prescription L-thyroxin for years. For this study they simply included a selenium supplement. After three months they recorded an increase of 45% in serum selenium, a 21% increase in glutathione AND a reduction in thyroid antibodies by 76%. This is a huge positive shift. Upon withdrawal of the selenium alone, both serum selenium and glutathione levels promptly fell with a marked increase in her antibodies.[39]

Here are the primary nutrients that successfully increase glutathione levels both systemically and locally around the thyroid. You will notice that oral glutathione is not listed because once it hits the stomach it becomes mostly inactive.

~ Selenium methionine; this was already mentioned in the section on nourishing the thyroid gland.

~ N-Acetyl Cysteine at 1,000mg twice daily. This has been proven to increase glutathione levels. If you suspect you have absorbed heavy metals from say dental amalgams then start more slowly at 250mg twice daily. NAC does mobilize and helps to secrete heavy metals.

Taking oral glutathione under the tongue will be absorbed directly into the blood stream through the small capillary bed. This area under the tongue and the rest of the mouth and cheeks are rich in lymphatic vessels. When glutathione is absorbed through mouth and cheeks it flows through these lymph channels and passes around and through the thyroid gland.

~ Douglas Labs is the only company I know of at this time that makes a sublingual L-Glutathione.

This product does contain a little N-Acetyl Cysteine and mannitol, which for some people causes a little irritation. Just bite the small tablet into a kind of paste and swish it back and forth under the tongue and around the inside of the cheeks. Take one table twice daily.

Another route to getting glutathione into the area of the thyroid is through the use of topical glutathione. I have specially formulated a liquid, medical grade, DMSO product that includes 2,000mg of pure glutathione. DMSO simply acts as a carrier to facilitate the absorption of glutathione directly into the area surrounding the thyroid gland.

Omega III oils should also be included since they have proven anti-inflammatory effects. Nordic Naturals has been manufacturing fish oil products for decades and their standards are among the highest.

Repair Thyroid Cells

Many of the nutrients already covered will help repair damaged thyroid cells. There is another product I've found useful. We never know how well the thyroid may be able to actually regenerate new thyroid cells but we need to repair those that remain intact in order to maximize their thyroid hormone production.

~ Mixed EFA's from Biotics Research. It contains Walnut, Hazelnut, Sesame, and Apricot Kernel oils.

Use a tablespoon a day with food.

Kick the Gluten Habit

Celiac disease is an autoimmune inflammatory condition of the small intestine. Gluten found in foods such as wheat, oats, rye and barley is the antigen or molecule that stimulates the activity of white blood cells leading to this inflammation which leads to problems with nutrient absorption and other intestinal symptoms.

Celiac disease has been connected with numerous conditions including Type I Diabetes, Addison's disease, hypo and hyperparathyroidism, deficiencies of vitamins and minerals including D, iron and zinc, fertility problems, hypogonadism in men, and autoimmune thyroid disease (AITD).[40]

One study of 423 Sardinian children with celiac disease were assessed for AITD and studied over a 10 year period. At the beginning of the study some of the children already had AITD while others developed AITD during the 10 years of the study. In the end, 70 of the 423 children had AITD.[41] I suspect that after the 10 year study, many of these children and adolescents went on to develop AITD over their lifetime.

In one study out of Italy, they found a correlation between celiac disease and selenium deficiency. They considered this deficiency to be "an important direct factor of thyroidal damage in the development of AITD."[42]

There is a difference between Celiac disease and a gluten intolerance or sensitivity but this is too detailed to cover right now. Just know that gluten intolerance is suspected to afflict about 12% of our general population[4] while Celiac affects approximately 1%. Even though 12% doesn't sound like much, that's about 42 million people in the U.S. alone.

I've seen a very high number of Hashimoto's patients recover much more quickly, in both symptoms and improved lab tests, by avoiding gluten foods when compared with patients who were unable to follow the avoid gluten guideline.

Just to give you one example of how severe a gluten intolerance can be, there was a 48 year old woman with severe Hashimoto's symptoms. She followed many of my recommendations but still wasn't improving all that much. This was during a time when I didn't understand the link between Hashimoto's and gluten. After several months we decided to try the gluten free diet.

She returned in a month with a huge smile on her face. She felt so much better than before and all we had changed was her diet. Everything else had remained the same. For the next 2 months she continued to improve. She was back to her old self.

On a future visit she came in with a remarkable story. During a meal with her family she had cut off a pat from a stick of butter and noticed a small crumb stuck to it. It had likely come off of her son's knife since he had just finished buttering his wheat toast. She thought nothing of it. Later that day she had a huge aggravation of her previous symptoms. This taught me a lesson about people who are highly sensitive. They cannot take even a crumb.

I also know that when people avoid gluten their thyroid antibodies are much lower than when they eat gluten. This has been proven several times. I was sure that one woman had Hashimoto's based on her fluctuating TSH levels but she showed me the negative results from her TPO antibody test. I wondered about her nutrition and if her diet was gluten free. She had been off gluten for years since she had a history of intestinal problems that had greatly improved with her new diet.

I asked her to repeat the TPO antibody test after eating gluten for two days. This time her antibodies were elevated. Why would I want to know if she had antibodies? Because I wanted to be certain she could take iodine and iodide without activating her Hashimoto's when starting on higher doses.

So I hope you understand how important it is to avoid gluten. I usually tell people to avoid it for 2 weeks which for many people, is psychologically possible. I then have them challenge gluten by taking it a couple of times after the two week period to witness their reaction first hand. So often this experience is very convincing and they realize that gluten must be avoided if they are to recover their health.

I cannot say if the avoidance of gluten will be a lifetime dietary change or not. Once your antibodies are down and you've passed through Phase II of the treatment program you can have your TPO antibodies checked after eating gluten.

Avoiding gluten for many people requires a big commitment because wheat is so much a part of our culture. There are many books written on this subject which offer many alternatives to these grains.

Investigate other Causes of Symptoms

Every thyroid and Hashimoto's patient I've ever consulted with has had additional reasons for their symptoms. Here is a list of these other non-thyroid conditions that comingle with Hashimoto's symptoms.

Adrenal Fatigue

Our adrenals produce several hormones, one of them being cortisol. The insufficient production of cortisol can cause a variety of symptoms including fatigue, low blood pressure, dizziness upon standing, low blood sugar with the person having to eat often, eyes being sensitive to bright lights, and others.

Suboptimal production of cortisol is very common with Hashimoto's since this condition is a constant stress on our immune system. There are other causes of low cortisol production including chronic infections, unremitting stress, diets lacking specific nutrients including protein and essential fatty acids, lack of sleep, chronic pain and chronic inflammation to name a few.

General fatigue and malaise are also common complaints of low thyroid hormones and low blood sugar and it can be difficult to differentiate between these and low cortisol levels.

When a person begins to experience fatigue due to low thyroid hormone production it's their adrenals which must take up the slack. The long term result of this is eventual adrenal exhaustion and suboptimal production of cortisol.

On the other hand if the person begins to experience even mild adrenal deficiency with lower cortisol production this will compromise the conversion of the thyroid hormone T4 to the activating T3 hormone and reduce the ability of the T3 to bind to their receptors inside the nucleus of our cells.

I often find that I cannot treat a thyroid condition without also optimizing a person's cortisol levels.

The first thing to do is to test your cortisol levels. This is a little difficult through the traditional blood test. Since cortisol levels change rapidly with stress, the setting of a lab and the pain of the blood draw will provoke the adrenals to secrete cortisol.

Even though a person may have low cortisol reserves, this sudden spike due to the stress of the draw will cause their results to appear normal within the lab's reference range. This gives the false impression that everything is fine.

For this reason some physicians prefer to check a saliva cortisol levels. This is a simple test done at home in a more relaxed setting and thus removes the variable of stress, resulting in a more accurate reading.

If a person has general fatigue throughout the day then two saliva samples are enough with one collection in the morning and the second in the evening.

If their energy fluctuates a lot throughout the day and they even have symptoms of agitation and anxiety (possibly elevated cortisol) then they should collect another sample mid-day.

If there's trouble with insomnia or difficulty with falling to sleep then a night time sample before bed is important.

So what's next? What can be done if a person has low cortisol levels?

First of all become educated. One of my favorite books ever is *Safe Uses of Cortisol* by Dr. William Jefferies, M.D. His research and clinical practice began when cortisol as a prescription was first introduced in the late 1940's and his publication covers 5 decades of research and clinical cases.

Dr. Jefferies' primary emphasis was to understand the difference between physiological and pharmacological dosing of cortisone and that health and vitality require normal or optimal levels of cortisol production. It's when you enter the arena of pharmacological (high) dosing of cortisone that the negative effects show up. These effects are the reason why cortisone has such a bad reputation.

His publication clearly explains how to dose cortisol in a way that maintains optimal, health-promoting levels.

Second, get plenty of sleep and rest, at least 8 hours per night. If you wake up and cannot get back to sleep it could be a sign of low cortisol since cortisol prevents us from going into hypoglycemia. If we fall into hypoglycemia we wake up in a fight or flight mode with all the accompanying adrenal hormones including adrenaline.

In this case be sure to eat something before retiring, something that takes a while for the body to break down into glucose. This would be any kind of animal protein since it also contains fat which is slow to be metabolized. Nuts such as almonds will also help to maintain a more normal blood sugar through the night.

Just to note, another common reason to wake up at night and thus disrupting the night time production of cortisol by the adrenals in preparation for the next day, is needing to urinate. The most common cause of this is a systemic Candida problem. This is covered in another section.

Next, avoid waiting too long between meals. Be sure not to go longer than 3 hours after eating before you eat or snack again. When your blood sugar begins to fall the only way to stop it is to either eat something or for your adrenals to produce cortisol which converts fat and protein into glucose. So every time your blood sugar drops and you don't eat, you are straining your adrenals.

Do not exercise on an empty stomach since this will lead to low blood sugar. In fact I recommend to people to avoid aerobic exercise if they have even mild adrenal deficiency. They may feel better afterwards but in the long run they are just making things worse. Using weights is preferable yet still, not on an empty stomach.

Dr. Jefferies comments on the effect of tobacco and caffeine upon the adrenals. From a couple of research papers, Dr. Jefferies' thinking is that both of these substances stimulate the production of ACTH, the hormone that triggers the adrenals to release more cortisol.

Caffeine also stimulates the conversion of a specific form of fat (glycogen) into glucose, thus raising blood sugar levels.

For tobacco, I suggest the practice of not inhaling the smoke as deeply and to switch to American Spirit to avoid the chemicals added to the more commercial brands. Every time we introduce chemicals and toxins into our system our adrenals go into an alarm state.

For caffeine, I suggest introducing decaffeinated beans when making your coffee. For some of you suffering from severe fatigue and having to push through the day with the use of caffeine, you will likely need to start mixing decaf with regular coffee beans otherwise you will go through caffeine withdrawals.

Using a B complex with at least 250mg of B5 or Pantothenic Acid can help.

If your physician agrees you can use small physiological doses of cortisol taking around 5mg three to four times daily with food. My experience with this approach has mirrored the clinical results of Dr. Jefferies. Of course if your physician has not read *Safe Uses of Cortisol* their response will most often be quite negative. Their response is only because of ignorance so don't take it personally. If you have the money present him or her with a copy of Dr. Jefferies book. It has the potential to change their practice.

You also have the option of using an adrenal glandular which contains the hormone cortisol. If you want to try this approach the product I recommend is Cytozyme AD from Biotics Research. The usual dose is to take 2 between 3-4 times daily at the beginning of a meal.

The adrenal cortex, the part of the adrenal gland which makes cortisol, has the highest concentrations of vitamin C of all the body's tissues. It is suspected that this vitamin plays an important role in the production of cortisol. This may be one reason why vitamin C is so important to prevent and fight infections since cortisol is essential for mobilizing and activating your immune system. When people can afford it, I always recommend the natural food form of C since it contains other important cofactors including copper. Innate Response makes a high potency vitamin C product made from food with each tablet containing the approximate equivalent of three oranges.

Allergies in General

Allergic reactions can be due to a wide variety of antigens found in foods, the environment, cosmetics, our spouse….eh, just kidding. Food allergies are reduced by eating a more hypoallergenic diet, one free of additives, preservatives and colorings. There are a number of foods that can cause allergic reactions. These include dairy products, corn, eggs, grains, peanuts, soy products, shellfish and others.

Sometimes allergic reactions are immediate and the person knows which foods to avoid. Yet sometimes, in fact most of the time, allergic reactions are delayed making it more difficult to trace which food has caused a set of less acute or vague symptoms. There are blood tests to help uncover these delayed reactions to antigens yet they are a bit pricy. Take a look at the Brenaman Hypoallergenic Diet as another approach to investigate delayed food allergies.

For allergies to cosmetics consider using a line that is chemical free and hypoallergenic. I know this is not a guarantee since cosmetic companies are totally unaccountable for what they list on their labels. Their ingredients can even include hormones. There are some lines of organic cosmetics with up to 98% organic ingredients.

In general allergies are a sign of weak adrenals which must be addressed. Yet many seasonal and environmental allergies can be improved by taking an herb called Stinging Nettles or Urtica dioca. I've been using Eclectic Institute products for over 25 years and have always been pleased with their quality. They make a wildcrafted, freeze dried Nettles with around 300mg per capsule. This has always been effective. It does help to open a couple of capsules into a cup, add boiling water and let it steep for 5 minutes.

Allergies to Molds

I made this a separate heading because this allergy is extremely common yet people are generally oblivious of the severe negative effects molds have upon their health.

Two people can live in the same moldy house with one feeling fine while the other can be so sick they are almost bedridden.

A person can feel much better when away on vacation. They think it's because there's less stress or because of a healthier climate yet when they return home they fall right back into their familiar set of symptoms. Their living and work environments need to be investigated for molds.

If you suspect an allergy to mold then you need to investigate areas of your home where mold is most common. Some people already know where the mold is but they don't believe it has any effect upon their condition. Do not be fooled. Molds spread through the air of the entire home and overwhelm the immune system.

With mold allergies a person must have a sensitivity or predisposition in order to have a reaction. Most of the time the medical history of people who've developed allergies to molds is riddled with the use of excess antibiotics, oral contraceptives, low-fat, high-carbohydrate, sugar-filled diets, having never been breast fed (Colostrum), and often with a history of having lived in a home full of obvious molds. They react to molds in every form including minimal levels of molds in their home, perfumes, leftover foods, corn, nuts, soy, products from corn fed animals, and others.

Environmentally these people <u>must</u> clean up their living space. This means getting rid of everything that has molds, including moldy carpets and even plants due to molds in the soil. They must also clean up cluttered and musty basements. People who live in regions where there are more severe seasonal changes often store their line of winter and summer clothes in the basement and these absorb molds. Usually basements, even clean basements, will have molds. It's important to avoid spending time in basements, being sure that the door leading to the basement remains closed and that the duct system does not draw air from the basement into the rest of the house. Ducts that draw air from the basement must be closed. Be sure to check if there is a humidifier in your heating system.

I had purchased a two-story home with beautiful gardens and a patio where patients could wait for their appointment. It was one of my dreams to practice in a beautiful, less clinical setting. We were painting and arranging the interior in preparation for our clinic's open house when my two employees started having a slight cough and sinus congestion. Since they had both been in good health for the last year and because they came down with the symptoms at the same time, I investigated the heating and duct system.

I found a rectangular pan in the ducts that was normally filled with water for humidifying the air traveling through the ventilation system to all the rooms. This pan was full of black-brown mold. Once this was removed, within a day both women were back to health.

If possible, remove worn carpets since most of the time they have been cleaned and shampooed annually. Cleaning carpets is usually fine as long as two things are taken into account.

First, molds form when carpets remain moist for too long. If you are planning to have your carpets cleaned, they must be thoroughly vacuumed. Any dirt or dust in the carpets will absorb moisture and extend drying time. Most carpet cleaning businesses use industrial vacuum cleaners in preparation for cleaning. The typical home vacuum cleaners are not powerful enough.

Second, do not have your carpets cleaned in the winter since windows will remain closed trapping dampness, which slows down the drying process. If you live in an area with humid summers then clean carpets in the seasons when there is less humidity and windows can remain open for better circulation.

Once you've addressed carpets and removed anything from the house that is moldy, the next step is to clean moldy areas of the house. I suggest if you are allergic to have someone else use bleach diluted in water to kill surface molds that are visible. These are often areas with a history of water leaks or where molds have collected in damp areas (basements, windowsills, etc.). Use a bristle brush to go deep into wood and concrete. You will not get results with diluted bleach applied to carpets. Take your rugs in for steam cleaning.

The next step is to clear molds from the house in general. This is done through the use of an ozone generator that can be purchased or rented. I suggest doing one room at a time by opening all cupboard and closet doors, exposing any areas you know to be moldy, and closing the room off from the rest of the house. Run towels under doors to contain the ozone gas and run the generator for 10-12 hours per room. Ozone will irritate the lungs so avoid breathing it. Once the room has been ozonated, open all of the windows and leave the room for half an hour.

There is a product I've found to be very effective for reducing a person's sensitivity to molds. I have witnessed changes in people, physically and psychologically, including the clearing of depression, apathy and anxiety that are often aggravated by mold exposure.

The product is called *Mold, Yeast & Dust* by BioAllers. It is a homeopathic preparation of various molds including Aspergillus, Penicillium, glandulars, herbs, Candida Albicans, dust, etc. I've treated many people with Penicillin allergies and haven't had a single person react unfavorably to the homeopathic preparation of

Penicillin in this product. Start with a drop at a time and work up to the product's recommended dose.

Even though people experience an improvement in their symptoms using this product it is not a substitute for cleaning up their environment.

So that's the external approach to treating mold allergies. The internal approach has to do with altering and improving the ecology of the intestines. This is all about increasing the population of good bacterial flora while reducing the internal mold or fungus. This subject is covered in another section on Candida.

Blood Sugar

Every symptom that we experience with Hashimoto's is accentuated by high and low levels of blood sugar. By simply maintaining blood sugar within a fairly optimal range throughout the day a person can feel 20-30% better from this alone.

The first step is to select foods that help to stabilize blood sugar and for this reason you should know a little about how your body regulates blood glucose. I am not talking about calories here at all. I am talking about feeling better through eating foods that maintain optimal blood glucose levels.

When you eat any food, your blood sugar rises and this signals the release of a hormone called insulin. This hormone helps to move glucose out of the blood and into cells.

As glucose moves out of the blood stream and into your cells, glucose levels in the blood drop. This decline in blood glucose can be dramatic if too much insulin has been released. If too much insulin is released then too much glucose will leave the bloodstream and the person will experience a low blood sugar situation known as hypoglycemia. When this happens a number of internal alarms go off including the release of cortisol and adrenaline from the adrenals. This is not good for our immune system or our emotions, and for that matter, our adrenals. We are in a fight or flight mode.

Ideally we want to keep our blood sugar within the optimal range of 85 and 120 throughout the day.

The best way to regulate blood sugar is by selecting foods that do not cause great fluctuations. If a food converts to glucose quickly then our blood sugar will rise way above 120. This high blood sugar stimulates a lot more insulin release than were the blood sugar to rise to only 120. High blood sugar, with the corresponding high release of insulin, causes a rollercoaster of mood swings and physical symptoms.

If you eat nothing for 12 hours your blood sugar will reach a level which is pretty stable and well regulated. Testing your blood for glucose at this time indicates your fasting blood sugar. Then say you eat an Almond Joy candy bar. One Almond Joy has 24 grams of sugar in it. Since there are about 4.2 grams of sugar in a teaspoon, eating an Almond Joy is equivalent to eating about 6 teaspoons of sugar. That's a lot and so your blood sugar is going to rise considerably. If we tested your blood sugar about a half-hour after eating that delicious Almond Joy we'd find it quite elevated and likely well above 120.

Some foods create very high blood glucose levels while the affect of others is more moderate. We have a pretty good idea about how rapidly various foods convert to sugar by measuring blood sugar before and after eating a food. In this way foods are rated for what is called their glycemic (glucose) index.

Sugar has a glycemic index of 100. Here are a few other foods with their ratings. Naturally if we want to stabilize our blood sugar we want to select foods which have a lower rating.

Breakfast Cereals
Corn flakes	92
Rice Krispies	82
Shredded Wheat	75
Instant Cream of Wheat	74
Cream of Wheat	66

Quick Oats	66
Muesli	43
All Bran with Fiber	38

Vegetables
Parsnips	97
Pumpkin	75
Beets	64
Corn	60
Carrots	49
Lettuce	10
Cabbage	10
Broccoli	10

Sweeteners
Pancake Syrup	76
Jams	65
Honey	55
Fructose	19

Grains
Instant White Rice	87
White Rice	72
Brown Rice	55
Barley	25

Bread
French Baguette	95
Bagel	72
Whole meal Rye	58
Stone Ground Wheat	53

Beans
Kidney Beans Canned	52
Lentils	29
Kidney Beans Dried	28

Potatoes
Instant Mashed	86
Baked Potato	85
New Potato	57
Yams	37

Because of how slowly we digest and metabolize animal proteins into glucose, they do not normally elevate blood sugar above 120 and are therefore not included in this list.

Also we seldom have a single food for a meal. So as soon as we add another food to our plate, or even some fat such as butter to our bread, the speed of absorption is slowed and our blood glucose won't rise as quickly or as high.

As an example, comparing a non-fat ice cream with a whole fat ice cream with all their other ingredients being the same, the low fat will have a higher glycemic index because it is absorbed more quickly. Fat slows absorption.

The idea then is to keep blood sugar within an optimal range by choosing low glycemic foods and by not skipping meals.

Candida

The ecology of the intestines is a vast subject so I need to focus on one condition that is very common among people with

Hashimoto's and the general population. I'd say that approximately 80% of the people I consult with have this problem to some degree.

The condition of Candidiasis (chronic Candida albicans infection) is a fungal infection or overgrowth of fungus in the intestines. Candida is normally found in the gut, yet if its growth is out of control it can lead to a wide variety of symptoms including the intensification of Hashimoto's symptoms. Here is a very brief list of frequently experienced symptoms.

- ~ Fatigue
- ~ Sadness and depression
- ~ Weight gain
- ~ Fluid retention
- ~ Indigestion
- ~ Skin problems including eczema and psoriasis
- ~ Foggy brain with difficulty concentrating
- ~ Headaches
- ~ Frequent urination
- ~ Vaginal discharge with itchiness
- ~ Cravings for sweets and starches

An overgrowth of Candida results primarily from the abuse or prolonged use of antibiotics including tetracycline for acne, birth control pills, and a high-sugar, low-fat, high-carbohydrate diet. People who were not breastfed also have an increased risk of Candida overgrowth.

Unless this gastrointestinal fungal infection is greatly reduced, Hashimoto's and other thyroid symptoms may only improve by 60-75%. It's not until Candida levels are minimized that a person will truly feel themselves again.

There are many books written about Candida. A couple of titles I recommend are the following;

~ The Yeast Connection by Dr. William Crook, M.D.
~ Chronic Candidiasis by Dr. Michael Murry, N.D.

In brief, my approach is four-fold.

1. Clean up the external environment of molds.
2. Follow a specific dietary plan which removes foods containing molds while avoiding foods which feed the Candida. Candida loves sugar and starch. You may have heard them whisper, "Let's get some Krispy Kremes..."
3. Improve the bacterial flora of the gut.
4. Use herbs and other supplements to lower the Candida population.

Here is a list of the products I've found to be effective.

~ Colostrum, to improve bacterial flora. This is kind of like the soil in which other good bacteria will implant. Symbiotics makes Colostrum Plus which I've had good results with.

~ There are many acidophilus products on the market which can be found locally. The only precaution or disadvantage of using acidophilus is its sensitivity to the hydrochloric acid (HCl) produced in the stomach. The product we keep on our shelves is one from Thorne Research, called Bacillus Coagulans. It contains a particular acid producing, beneficial bacteria which resists being digested by hydrochloric HCl.

~ Grapefruit Seed Extract (GSE) is one anti-Candida product. This comes in both a capsule and liquid form. The capsule form is used to reduce the Candida population in the small intestines. The liquid form is for those who have a white or gray coating on their tongue. In their case the Candida has migrated up into the stomach, esophagus and mouth.

~ SF722 from Thorne Research is another. It contains an extract from the castor bean.

~ Tanalbit is a third anti-Candida product made from plant tannins. It is also considered an anti-inflammatory as well as an anti-parasitic.

There's a reason for listing three products for reducing Candida levels. This is because Candida can develop resistant strains just like bacteria can become resistant to antibiotics. This has been my experience with people who have been on an anti-Candida product for years and are still suffering. Their Candida has become resistant and thus becomes more difficult to treat.

To avoid this you need to go through at least 2 different anti-Candida products and possibly three just to be sure. Finish one product and then go on to the next. Start slowly with the first product otherwise you'll experience a large die-off of the yeast and feel much worse. You don't need this. Take it slow at first.

I cannot tell you how many caps of each anti-Candida product to take since their strengths vary, and each person's condition is different. I recommend starting slowly and ending up somewhere around twice what the manufacturer recommends.

It requires a bit of experimenting to sense what dose of the anti-Candida product is best. Usually a person feels a slight stomach upset but they sense feeling better physically, and their mind feels a lot clearer.

Then there's the diet. Below is a list of foods to avoid and foods to include. The books I've mentioned will give more details though they differ slightly in their dietary suggestions.

Foods to Eat

Proteins; this includes any form of protein such as eggs, fish, red meat, lamb, pork, chicken, turkey, sardines, etc. Try to include organic and stay away from corn fed if possible.

Veggies; the idea here is to eat vegetables with the least amount of starch in them. Candida loves sugar and starch. Vegetables with low starch are those that grow above the ground such as lettuce, spinach, chard, celery, cucumbers, green & red peppers, Brussels sprouts, etc. Vegetables that grow on and under the ground have a higher starch content and are more likely to raise the blood sugar. The occasional sweet potato, carrot or squash is OK.

Fruit; eat sparingly of any juicy fruit such as apples, peaches, pears, plums and grapes. Do not eat more than a handful a day. Avocados are in this category but can be eaten in addition to your handful of fruit since they do not contain sugar. Jams made from 100% fruit without any added sugars or artificial sweeteners are OK in small amounts.

Nuts, Seeds & Oils; I prefer it if people can stick with almonds and almond butter. Oils to use are cold pressed olive and coconut oils. Good quality cultured butter can be included as well.

Legumes; beans and lentils are good even though they have a high starch content. Best to sprout them first before cooking but this takes some devotion. I recommend taking them not more than 3 to 4 times weekly.

Dairy Product Substitutes; milks made from nuts and grains such as almonds and rice are fine but select the ones with the lowest grams of glucose or sugar.

Whole Grains; grains do convert to glucose and need to be used sparingly, preferably in small amounts at a meal. Brown rice, amaranth, quinoa, and millet are the ones to select from. Even whole grain gluten free pastas should be eaten sparingly since these are refined and processed.

Whole Grain Breads; You can include yeast and gluten free whole grain breads. You can toast the bread, add some cultured butter and almond spread, and a little unsweetened 100% fruit jam.

Foods to Avoid

Sugars and Foods High in Sugar; avoid foods and drinks that contain sugar in all forms. Avoid honey, molasses, maple syrup, date sugar and turbinado sugar. Of course avoid foods with artificial sweeteners. Fruits to be avoided are bananas, melons, canned fruits, bottled fruit juices, and citrus (lemons and limes are OK). You can use Stevia in small amounts.

Packaged & Processed Foods; move towards a healthier diet by avoiding canned, bottled, boxed and other packaged and processed foods such as bakery goods, mustards, ketchup, Worcestershire, accent, monosodium glutamate (this is an insidious ingredient, hiding in all kinds of foods, especially dressings), BBQ sauces, etc.

Dairy Products; this means any product made from cow's milk. For now it also includes products from goat's milk though goats will be the first to reintroduce when your Candida levels are down.

Yeast and Mold Containing Foods; corn, popcorn, corn oil, fermented products (cider, soy sauce, tamari, miso soup, vinegars), malt products, processed meats (sausage, hot dogs, corned beef, pastrami), mushrooms and fungi, tempeh, peanuts, old nuts, and, unless they are immediately refrigerated, no leftovers.

Alcohol; alcohol in all forms, yet a dry red or white wine, 2-4 ounces, taken only with food, not on an empty stomach, a few times per week is OK.

Acid Producing Foods; coffee, chocolate and tomato paste.

This is pretty much the nutritional program for lowering Candida in the gut. Usually the reduction of Candida to somewhat normal levels requires 6 to 12 weeks. When can a person say they are free from Candida and return to a normal diet? This really depends upon how severe a person's infection is yet a person usually knows when it's time.

People ask this question at the beginning, "Will I be on this diet forever? Will I ever be able to eat sugar and pastries again?" Yet what happens to almost everyone is that the nutritional program shifts their cravings and causes them to become more sensitive about the effect foods have upon their energy and moods. They realize the value of their health and they consciously choose to not slip back into their old eating habits.

It is common for people's desire for sweets to become much less. When they read through the list of foods to avoid they moan and shake their heads. "I'll never be able to follow this." But within

10-14 days they are feeling better and their sweet tooth is much less.

The thing is to just get started. Clear your kitchen of the foods you must avoid and then take one meal and one day at a time. The first seven days are a little rough with the die off of yeast, but with some obvious good days you'll begin to experience a sense of hope and improved health.

Drink lots of water and be sure your bowels are moving well. You want to excrete the Candida waste as quickly as possible.

Cholesterol & Health

For those of you who are vegetarians or if you believe that protein makes you fat I ask you to keep an open mind for a few minutes.

I have practiced for 27 years and the most difficult category of people to treat are those deficient in proteins and cholesterol. This is also true for people taking lipid lowering prescriptions where their cholesterol goes below 150.

For some people, and certainly not the majority, blood levels of cholesterol can become elevated from eating too many saturated fatty foods. Yet I have seen cholesterol levels in the 300's with vegetarians. I believe the approach of reducing cholesterol rich foods to the bare minimum is a hazard to people's health.

There needs to be a shift in our attitude about cholesterol since it plays a vital role in our health;

~ It is the major component of plasma membranes that surround every cell of your body. The health of every cell is dependent upon cholesterol's protective and fluid nature.

~ Bile is made from many ingredients including cholesterol and bile is essential for the absorption of essential fatty acids, lipids and oil soluble vitamins. Biotics Research makes a digestive enzyme called Beta Plus which includes Ox Bile extract to improve the absorption of essential fatty acids.

~ Vitamin D production from UV exposure requires the cholesterol molecule.

~ Cholesterol is the precursor or backbone of all the adrenal hormones including cortisol.

~ All male and female hormones (estrogens, progesterone, testosterone, etc.) require cholesterol for their production.

~ Low serotonin leads to aggressive, violent and suicidal behavior. Low cholesterol levels are linked to low serotonin in males.

~ The coating around certain nerves known as myelin is rich in cholesterol. The breakdown of this myelin sheath is found in Multiple Sclerosis and Diabetes.

Maintaining optimal cortisol levels with Hashimoto's is extremely important. Cortisol has anti-inflammatory properties and helps to interrupt the vicious cycle of over-reactive white blood cells and the release of thyroid cell debris due to cell destruction.

It is very common for people with Hashimoto's to have low adrenal function and low cortisol. Low cortisol is often due to decades of chronic inflammation and having to compensate for the chronic fatigue that accompanies low thyroid hormones.

Animal protein whether lean or fatty not only provides the adrenals with the cholesterol they need to make cortisol but also helps to maintain more optimal blood sugar levels. Fattier foods help to maintain normal blood sugar in order to avoid hypoglycemia or low blood sugar. Hypoglycemia strains the adrenals adding to chronic adrenal fatigue.

I clearly remember one 52 year old gentleman with complaints of fatigue. All his lab tests were normal except his blood sugar and cholesterol were on the low side. His employer was a very well known motivational speaker who had recovered his health through adopting a strict vegetarian diet.

This man, because of his employment, had taken on this same attitude about nutrition. I told him that his labs indicated the need for more protein in his diet and to consider including a steak and other forms of protein. His eyes lit up. When I saw him a month later his energy had returned.

Another gentleman in his late 40's had the same complaint but was a little less flexible with the idea of including a steak. So I suggested yoghurt from whole milk, which included more fat. He called the office in three days to thank me for the suggestion. He had noticed an improvement within 24 hours from this simple change in his diet.

When I first started my practice the upper normal of the lab's reference range for cholesterol was 250. It's now been reduced to 200 and the pharmaceutical companies are making bundles from the sale of lipid lowering drugs.

Remember that on a lab test the cholesterol level includes the various forms of cholesterol including the protective form, HDL, or High Density Lipoproteins. But as soon as most doctors see any cholesterol level above 200 they start talking about a prescription, partly believing this is the practice of preventative medicine. Generally they have forgotten that there's an essential need for optimal levels of cholesterol and have also forgotten to ask the question, "Why is this person's cholesterol above the 'normal' range?"

There are always reasons, one of which is low thyroid hormone levels. They have also forgotten that dietary habits have little to do with high cholesterol unless a person is eating a lot of the bad fats or trans, hydrogenated (oxidized) fats often found in packaged goods such as chips, pretzels, cookies, fast food, shortenings and some margarine brands. They are also found in some brands of peanut butter. Because the body can't break them down, these trans fats attach to the arteries and may result in plaque formation, which can be linked to heart disease, diabetes, breast cancer and asthma, as well as other illnesses.

I recently received a lab test that was done at the Hippocrates' Institute in Florida where clients undergo programs for cleansing, eating mostly raw foods and avoiding animal protein. This lady's lab report showed their upper normal reference range was 170. Apparently this institution has the same mindset that cholesterol is bad. How unfortunate for those clients who already have progesterone and cortisol deficiencies.

Part of helping people to recover their health is teaching them to listen to their instincts. Questioning the programming we receive through our media is a big step and exercising our intuition around eating whole foods which our ancestors ate is another.

Your body is like a small laboratory. You know how you feel after eating certain foods. If you feel physically better and more energetic and your mental focus is clearer, then you know. If you feel more tired and foggy, then avoid the food. It's up to you.

Chronic Infections

This subject is very important. There are two types. The first type causes symptoms which the person is usually aware of while the second type is usually hidden or silent and the person may experience only a general sense of chronic fatigue.

The first type is fairly easy to remedy with lots of immune supporting nutrients such as vitamins A, E and C as well as the minerals zinc and selenium and a number of herbs such as Echinacea, myrrh, garlic and cayenne. All these ingredients can be found in a single product from Eclectic Institute called OptiBiotic. I've used this for about 25 years with amazing success for even obstinate Streptococcal infections. OptiBiotic is their professional label name. The retail label name is VitaBiotic which has identical ingredients.

Watch for recurring throat infections especially when a person has had their tonsils removed. These infections are especially nasty because bacteria have become imbedded in the scar tissue which formed as a result of the surgery. The infection remains since there's very little blood circulation in scar tissue so the white cells can't get in.

Another includes sinus infections. These cavities, which are sort of external to the body, make it very difficult for our immune system to put up a good fight. These often require the use of a Neti pot to wash out these cavities using saline, diluted hydrogen peroxide, diluted Hydrastis or goldenseal, and diluted iodine.

You need to also use an old naturopathic treatment called hydrotherapy. This involves applying alternating hot and cold water to the face and sinuses.

Stand with your head over the sink and cup hot water using a washcloth in the palms of your hands. Bring this hot water to the face and hold it there. Repeat this for about a minute until the face is nice and red. Then turn the cold tap on and do the same, continuing to bring cold water to the face and sinuses. Do this for about a minute as well.

Repeat this cycle, hot and cold, three times. By the second or third cycle you should begin to experience sinus drainage. Blowing your nose will help to dislodge mucous. This can be done twice daily. If you are using a Neti pot then do this after the hydrotherapy.

It's very important to resolve these infections because they drain the vitality of our immune system as well as the hormone cortisol from our adrenals. I suggest using the VitaBiotic for any infection, both acute and chronic. This product does contain a pretty high dose of vitamin A and therefore should be used with caution if you are pregnant. A pregnant woman should not be taking more than 10,000 units of vitamin A per day.

The chronic silent infections are different because people are usually not aware of them. The most common location is a root canalled tooth. Another location might be any scar or previous surgery. These should be investigated by a knowledgeable health professional.

Halogens

These earth elements include fluoride, chlorine and bromine which are found in our water supply, toothpastes, swimming pools, hot tubs, cleaning materials, breads and soft drinks. Watch out for bromine in brominated sodas, sedatives, cough medicines, spa pools, hair permanent solutions and brominated vegetable oils. Read labels.

With Hashimoto's there's often a low concentration of iodine and iodide in the thyroid cells with a significant increase in the concentration of bromine. The theory is that all halogens compete for entry into the thyroid. If iodide levels are low then bromine supersedes.

In Phase I it is very important to read labels and to exclude all the halogens including fluoride in toothpastes. In Phase II the introduction of iodine and iodide will help to excrete halogens from the body, especially from the thyroid.

It is somewhat common for a person to have skin eruptions when the reintroduce iodine and iodide. These eruptions may be from the excretion of halogens through the skin. These eruptions have been labeled both bromoderma and halogen acne. This skin reaction is temporary and can be improved by using products that focus on detoxification.

~ Biogenesis makes a great product, BioCleanse Plus

As I've already mentioned, saunas and anything that promotes sweating are very helpful as well.

Heavy Metals

The most common heavy metals I've found which interfere with thyroid function and delay the recovery from Hashimoto's are those found in dental amalgams.

Amalgams contain almost 50% elemental mercury with the remaining metals being silver, tin and copper. There is little disagreement about the toxic nature of mercury and the detrimental and destructive effects it has upon our cells, especially those of the neurological system.

Mercury is lipophilic, it loves lipids or fats. The membranes of our cells, including the thyroid cells are a double lipid, single protein matrix. Mercury can enter each and every cell and can readily cross over the blood brain barrier to enter brain cells.

One of the major secondary effects of mercury is that it depletes the body of antioxidants since they are used to clean up and remove heavy metals and other toxins. Glutathione is the premier antioxidant involved with heavy metal detoxification.

Hmmm...might there be a connection between heavy metals, the depletion of glutathione and selenium, and the inflammation of Hashimoto's Thyroiditis?

Almost all metals are solid at room temperature but not mercury. It is a liquid. Because of this unique quality pure mercury is used in thermometers because it expands and flows easily when warmed. Mercury is used in amalgams for this same reason. It adds pliability or plasticity to the mix of the other solid metals used in amalgams so it can be pressed into dental cavities of any shape.

The main problem with using mercury in amalgams is that mercury is volatile. You remember from science that matter has three possible states; solid, liquid and gas. Since mercury is a liquid at room temperature it will move in the direction of a gas when heated.

I vividly recall one presentation at a holistic medical conference given by a dentist. Every holistic dentist is in the business of replacing mercury amalgams with white or composite fillings. Because the drilling out of amalgam fillings creates so much friction and heat, which increases the vaporization of mercury, dentists are at great risk for mercury intoxication.

Over decades this dentist had become ill from this daily exposure to mercury. He recovered his health after going through a variety of detoxification protocols but still reacted when mercury vapors became elevated in his clinic. He needed to avoid these reactions and so he purchased an instrument to measure mercury vapors. When vapors reached a certain level in the clinic, a special air evacuation-ventilation system would kick in to clear the air.

So here's this holistic dentist with his amazing story of recovering from mercury intoxication holding in his hands this unit for measuring mercury vapors.

He asked for three volunteers who still had mercury fillings to come forward. He inserted a 4 inch straw into the intake valve of the unit and turned it on. Through this straw he drew air from within each volunteer's mouth, enabling him to read their levels of mercury vapor. I believe the measurements were in micrograms of mercury per liter of air. The ranges of these first three individuals were between 3 and 12 mcg/liter.

Then he gave each person a stick of chewing gum and they returned to their seats to have a chew.

After 10 minutes he asked them to return to the front. Now the lowest reading was 18 and the highest was in the 80's.

Without a doubt this demonstrated that the friction of chewing creates enough heat to cause the mercury in fillings to vaporize. And considering how many times per day we eat and also take hot drinks, we are obviously ingesting mercury.

It also helps to understand a bit about the measurement of mercury. Our Environmental Protection Agency (EPA) has set what they call a safe or acceptable level of exposure (ingestion) to mercury in our diet. They feel it's safe if our exposure does not exceed 0.1 mcg of mercury per kilogram of body weight in a given day.

www.epa.gov/mercury/exposure.html

It's not really clear to me how our agency came to believe that there's any safe exposure at all when it comes to mercury.

For a person weighting 150 pounds or 68kg this means their intake should not be more than 6.8mcg of mercury per day.

This may not seem like much since a mcg is 448 millionth of a pound, yet 1 mcg of mercury contains 3,000,000,000,000,000 atoms of mercury. This means that our EPA, which was established to protect us from environmental hazards, says that a 150 pound woman can safely ingest 20,400,000,000,000,000 atoms of mercury each day.

There is also an estimated range of how much mercury is ingested each day with mercury amalgams. It is between 3.5 and 21 mcg but I don't know how these figures were arrived at and this would certainly depend upon the number of fillings a person has. At any rate I am certain that having mercury fillings does not contribute to our health in any way.

Consider replacing your 'silver' amalgams with white ones. Some of your amalgams may be too large or too deep to replace and may need to remain. But remove what you can.

This procedure should be done by a qualified, mercury-free dentist. You will receive the quality of care and protection that this potentially dangerous procedure requires. Here is one site for more information. www.dentalwellness4u.com.

Increasing glutathione levels is extremely important whether or not you replace your fillings. I don't believe that glutathione is effective for pulling out mercury from fatty tissues, but it is for reducing harmful daily exposure.

The removal of the mercury that has accumulated in tissues over the years is a specialty unto itself and is called heavy metal chelation. This word simply means to grab onto the metal and to excrete it through the urine and stool. Chelation therapy is administered intravenously but there are some effective oral chelation products on the market.

Every company that manufactures oral chelation products will say theirs is the best and will give you lots of testimonials. But the only way to know for sure if a product is effective is through lab testing.

The procedure is to collect a sample of urine, ingest the chelating product in high doses and then to collect a second urine sample over the following hours. The two samples are compared and if the second sample has more heavy metals than the first then the product is effective.

This is a reliable and sensitive test and <u>anyone</u> selling a product for oral chelation should have these lab results to prove the effectiveness of their product. Companies know about these tests but have apparently chosen not to do them because their product is not that effective. And even when a company does present comparative lab results there is still no guarantee they are valid.

A group of investors had approached me to be the physician for a new venture. They had all the marketing connections through hundreds of magazines and they wanted to focus on oral heavy metal chelation. They had found a product online and the manufacturer included heavy metal urine results proving the effectiveness of their product.

My advice to this group was to first confirm the company's results by doing our own testing before they invested their money. So one of the investors, a patient and I followed the same testing procedures which the company had used. We each collected a morning urine sample upon rising. We then took the recommended amount of their oral heavy metal chelator and collected urine for the next six hours.

Neither our first urine sample or our second showed any heavy metals. Well, that's not exactly true. My first sample had tungsten, which I determined had come from the wok I had used the night before for cooking dinner. The only positive result from that experience was to rid my kitchen of all cooking utensils that were not stainless steel.

But I did eventually find one oral product which I've had great results with and the before and after urine analyses proved its effectiveness.

~ Waiora- liquid minerals formed deep within the earth's crust.

Use it as directed. Taking plenty of selenium and NAC will act synergistically with this product. In the case of Hashimoto's and other thyroid problems this liquid form is the best. Squeeze the drops under the tongue where it enters the blood stream and lymph vessels and then travels around and through the thyroid gland. Removing heavy metals is another way of cooling down white blood cell activity.

Progesterone & Estrogen

Many symptoms experienced by women with Hashimoto's may be related to low progesterone or what's called Estrogen Dominance, where the ratio of progesterone to estrogen (P:E) is low.

Symptoms of low progesterone are any of the following:

- ~ Acne
- ~ Anxiety
- ~ Depression
- ~ Foggy Thinking
- ~ Headaches
- ~ Insomnia Irritability
- ~ Lowered Sexual Desire
- ~ Mood Swings
- ~ Painful Breasts

~ Painful Joints

~ Poor Concentration

~ Swollen Breasts

~ Weight Gain

One reason why some of these symptoms are similar to low thyroid hormones is because thyroid cells have progesterone receptors, meaning that progesterone, when it couples with these receptors, stimulate thyroid cells to make thyroid hormones. Thus low progesterone can contribute to low thyroid hormone production.

And most women who consult about their condition of Hashimoto's do have low progesterone levels which have not been addressed by their physician. It is important for overall health to optimize progesterone levels.

Since we are interested in the free and available progesterone, what is unbound and able to leave the blood stream to circulate throughout the tissues, we use saliva hormone testing. The origin of saliva is lymph fluid which circulates throughout our tissues. Besides saliva being so easy to collect, we find this a very accurate way to assess progesterone levels.

Progesterone levels in the premenopausal woman do fluctuate through the cycle so we must be consistent with the days of collecting saliva. This collection is done on either days 19, 20 or 21 with day one being the first day of menstrual flow. For women past menopause their saliva is collected on any day.

This collection is done four times in one day, spitting saliva through a straw into a small plastic vial. Each kit comes with clear instructions on how to prepare for each collection.

Knowing the degree of progesterone deficiency helps to understand to what extent a woman's symptoms are likely due to a lack of this hormone and, to some extent, helps the clinician to prescribe the proper dosage.

There are different methods or routes of treating a progesterone deficiency. There are the 'natural' progesterone creams which can be very effective and bypass the need for a physician's prescription.

The line we most often recommend is from Emerita. Their bio-identical progesterone cream is called Pro-Gest which includes USP bio-identical progesterone with other natural ingredients, and is paraben free.

The prescriptions for bio-identical progesterone come in the form of creams, capsules and sublingual troches. Each has its special use.

The cream is applied to the areas of the body with the least amount of fat, usually the wrists, inner elbows, ankles, etc. This allows a steady stream of progesterone since the hormone is absorbed through the skin and then percolates into the lymph fluid which will eventually drain into the blood stream. This is normally used for the peri- and post-menopausal woman.

Capsules are swallowed with most of the progesterone broken down into another hormone called 17-hydroyprogesterone. This has a very relaxing effect, often bringing relief to headaches, insomnia and feelings of anxiety and agitation.

Troches are placed under the tongue and normally prescribed for women who are still menstruating, taking them once or twice daily on days 13 through 27. This approach respects the woman's normal monthly rhythm or cycle.

My experience with addressing Hashimoto's is that even though a person feels better when their thyroid inflammation and thyroid antibodies are lowered they still have some unresolved symptoms.

Low progesterone, or any low endocrine hormone for that matter, needs to be optimized.

For estrogen, some typical symptoms of inadequate estrogen are the following;

~ Anxiety

~ Depression

~ Dry Skin

~ Headaches

~ Heart Palpitations

~ Hot Flashes

~ Inability to Reach Orgasm

~ Lack of Menses

~ Memory Loss

~ Mood Swings

~ Night Sweats

~ Painful Intercourse

~ Vaginal Dryness

~ Vaginal Shrinkage

~ Yeast Infections

The approach for checking estrogen levels is the same as with progesterone, through the use of saliva hormone testing. Of course it's important to optimize estrogen levels for a number of health reasons yet estrogen should not be used without progesterone.

Bio-identical estrogen is another prescription item but can also be found in a non-prescription cream. The product we most often recommend for women preferring not to use a prescription is manufactured by Bio-Design called DermaEst which contains natural forms of progesterone, estriol, estradiol and estrone from wild yams. Its absorption is facilitated by MSM and is paraben free.

"You may encounter many defeats, but you must not be defeated. In fact, it may be necessary to encounter the defeats, so you can know who you are, what you can rise from, how you can still come out of it."

Maya Angelou

Phase II

Phase II is a lot simpler than Phase I. Now that TSH is below 1.0 we know that hydrogen peroxide production in thyroid cells has been minimized and with the use of antioxidants any inflammation has been even further reduced. The repair and regeneration of thyroid cells is underway. Your antibodies are also within normal limits.

We are now ready to activate the thyroid's production of thyroid hormones. Here are the objectives of Phase II.

~ Reintroduce iodine & iodide to activate thyroid hormone production and to saturate the body with these important essential elements.

~ Monitor antibodies to be certain they remain low.

~ Optimize thyroid hormone production by continuing to use all the supplements from Phase I.

~ Maintain low levels of thyroid inflammation through supplementation and dietary suggestions.

~ When we are assured that thyroid antibodies are not increasing we evaluate thyroid hormone production and metabolism (T4 to T3 conversion) through an extended thyroid lab panel.

Iodine & Iodide

During Phase I you've been taking all the nutrients your thyroid needs to make its hormones except for iodide because we didn't want to stimulate TSH production. Now the time has come to reintroduce it.

Yes, iodine and iodide will stimulate TSH production but we are not overly concerned with increasing hydrogen peroxide production at this point since levels of protective glutathione have greatly improved. Besides, we'll be introducing these iodide and iodine very slowly.

As TSH production is stimulated so will the production of thyroid hormones. This is an exciting time. But remember that you are likely taking a thyroid hormone and as your thyroid begins to produce its hormones you will likely have a little too much circulating thyroid hormones, experiencing some symptoms of hyperthyroidism. This direction is good because we are hoping that your thyroid will begin to make more of its own hormones so we don't want to stimulate TSH too much. This is another reason for introducing iodine and iodide slowly.

Remember that the half-life of T4 is seven days. About one-half of the T4 in the prescription you take today will still be circulating in your bloodstream seven days later. These hormones are added to those produced by your thyroid. Under normal circumstances TSH would start to drop if T4 gets a little too much, yet the iodine and iodide will continue to stimulate TSH production. This will not become a dangerous situation because we are slowly introducing. I will also explain how we can monitor thyroid hormone production in a moment.

We cannot use tablets of iodine and iodide because they are far too strong and concentrated. I suggest beginning with a liquid solution of Lugol's 2%, concentration of iodine and iodide.

Our starting dose of iodine and iodide will be 250mcg a day which is a very modest amount.

To calculate the dose of 250mcg you'll need to know a few things. One vertical drop (holding the dropper vertically and not horizontally) of Lugol's 2% is 2.5 mg of both iodine and iodide.

Translating 2.5 mg to mcg is 2,500 mcg. To get this 2,500 mcg drop down to 250 mcg requires dividing it by 10.

To do this put 20 tablespoons or a little over a cup (1.2 cups) of good quality water (not tap) into a jar that has a lid. Remove any Lugol's from the dropper and replace the dropper. Shake the bottle vigorously and then dispense two vertical drops into the jar. Secure the lid, shake it and take a tablespoon. This is 250 mcg of iodine and iodide.

One way to monitor hyperthyroid symptoms is through your resting heart rate. Resting means that you've not been physically active for the previous 15 minutes and you are not experiencing any anxiety. I suggest taking your pulse at night in bed.

Take your pulse for ½ minute and double it. This is your resting heart rate in beats per minute which normally ranges between 55 and 75. Begin a journal and record these readings.

One of the common signs of having too much circulating thyroid hormones is a rapid heart rate. There are others indications but this one is the most sensitive. So we'll use your heart rate to know if the combination of your thyroid prescription and the thyroid hormones produced by your thyroid is too much.

So here's a suggestion about how to take the Lugol's. It's rather simple. You'll be on a cycle of four days. Start with 1 tablespoon of the diluted Lugol's once daily for four days while monitoring your heart rate.

You will continue to increase the number of tablespoons every four days as long as your resting heart rate does not increase by more than 10 beats per minute. As long as you do not see an increase, this is the schedule for Lugol's 2%.

Days	Tablespoons	Iodine & Iodide	If you experience an increase in heart rate do not increase the number of tablespoons. Try to remain at the same number of tablespoons or reduce them by one or two. If you have any concerns about the effects of Lugol's stop taking it.
1-4	1	250mcg	
5-8	2	500mcg	
9-12	3	750mcg	
13-16	4	1,000mcg or 1mg	
17-20	6	1.5mg	
21-24	8	2mg	
25-28	10	2.5mg	
29 & on	12	3mg	

If your heart rate has not increased and you've been on the 3 mg dose for two weeks then it's time to check both TSH to see how much it has risen and thyroid antibodies to be sure they've not been reactivated. As long as your antibodies have not risen then everything is OK. TSH will likely be elevated above 2.0 but this is an expected result.

After your TSH and normal antibody lab results, I suggest running a complete thyroid hormone lab panel that I'll mention in just a bit. This panel will help to know how your thyroid is doing, if any adjustments need to be made, and how well you are converting T4 to T3.

The most common reaction to increasing Lugol's is an increase in heart rate. Remember that if your heart rate goes up by 10 beats per minute or more then do not increase Lugol's. Remain where you are.   If your heart rate remains elevated for another few days then it's time to reduce your thyroid prescription by a third to a quarter dose.

Remember, you always have the option of stopping Lugol's.

Realize that this increase in heart rate is telling you something, that your thyroid is making its own hormones. This is a very good sign.

Adjusting Thyroid Medication

Reducing your thyroid prescription by a third to a quarter dose will not have an immediate effect of lowering heart rate since the

T4 in the prescription has a half-life of 7 days. But it will start to come down in 3-5 days. Then when your heart rate has returned to where it was at the initial introduction of Lugol's, it's time to increase the number of tablespoons to the next level.

You will go through this same adjusting of your thyroid prescription every time your heart rate increases by 10 beats per minute.

This increase in heart rate is likely due to an increase in your thyroid's hormone production. However if you notice that as you increase the tablespoons of Lugol's that your heart rate is erratic, meaning that the rhythm is irregular, then the increase could be due to the activation of thyroid antibodies. Try getting to the stage of reducing your thyroid prescription at least once to see what happens. If it is remains erratic, then it's time to check your thyroid antibody levels.

I believe the above is pretty clear. If you don't have an increase in heart rate you continue increasing the number of tablespoons until you reach 3mg. If there is an increase in your heart rate you remain at the same number of tablespoons and reduce your medication. The idea is to reach 3mg of iodine and iodide while reducing the thyroid prescription to its minimum.

In either case, once you've reached the plateau of 3mg two weeks later you'll test TSH and thyroid antibodies. If your antibodies are normal then 2 weeks later you'll run the complete thyroid hormone panel.

You can also switch from the Lugol's to our product, IodoPlus-3 which is the same milligrams of iodine and iodide in a single capsule along with 400 mcg of selenium methionine. This is a one capsule a day formulation and any other intake of selenium should be discontinued.

Monitor with Lab Tests for Antibodies & TSH

If your antibodies become elevated in Phase II then you must return to Phase I for 4 weeks. Then have your antibodies and TSH rechecked. If they are low, then return to Phase II. This time you must introduce Lugol's more slowly than the first time.

You must also consider the following;

~ If you have not been strict with avoiding gluten then you'll need to be 100% gluten free.

~ If you have not done the heavy metal detoxification then use Waiora and consider finding a holistic dentist.

~ If you have not done the Candida treatment, then now's the
time.

~ If you have been applying the topical DMSO with
glutathione twice daily then go to four times daily.

~ Include vitamin C and consider the natural form (Innate
Response) taking a minimum of 4,000mg daily.

So let us say you are Hashimoto's free and you've have the results
from the complete thyroid hormone panel. What's the next step?

"I finally realized that being grateful to my body
was key to giving more love to myself."
Oprah Winfrey

Phase III

The optimization of thyroid hormones is the focus of this third phase.

Balancing Thyroid Hormone Levels

What I am about to cover is a bit more complex, yet very important to understand. This section will be a summary from my first book, *Low Thyroid Hormone Symptoms- 7 Causes & 7 Solutions.*

Even when your thyroid's production of T4 is perfect you can still suffer from low thyroid hormone symptoms. Here's why.

The lab test T4 (thyroxin) is an excellent way to assess thyroid health. If the thyroid is getting plenty of TSH stimulation this T4 should be around 8.5 or 9. This is ideal. The T4 lab test measures both the protein-bound T4 and the free or available T4 circulating in the blood.

Sometimes T4 can be highly bound leaving very little available. If it's bound it can't leave the blood stream and therefore can't be used. To find out how much of the Total T4 is bound we do the Free T4 lab test. If free or available T4 is low with a normal T4 then we know that too much of the T4 is bound. Highly bound T4 points to liver and, or, elevated estrogen and low progesterone.

But the Free T4 has very little to do with activating the body's metabolism. It must be converted to T3. This conversion is a very important step in optimizing thyroid hormone levels and requires various nutrients, especially selenium.[43]

Since T3 is what drives cell energy production and metabolism, it's a very important hormone to test. The Free T3 indicates how much of this hormone is able to leave the blood stream to do its thing.

If Free T4 is normal and Free T3 is low then there's a conversion problem. If both Free T4 and Free T3 are low then it may or may not be a conversion problem since Free T4 is required to make T3.

I know this may be a little too complex, but just so you know, whatever the reasons for low thyroid hormones there are solutions.

Low T4, as long as there's plenty of TSH, can be corrected by feeding the thyroid the nutrients it needs to produce its hormones.

Low Free T4, as long as Total T4 is normal, is corrected by improving liver function and balancing hormones.

Low Free T3, as long as there is plenty of Free T4, is corrected by improving liver function, taking plenty of selenium, and correcting any cortisol deficiency since this hormone is important for conversion.

And even when all the hormones (TSH, T4, Free T4 and Free T3) are optimal you can still have low thyroid hormone symptoms because of vitamin D and vitamin A deficiencies. Both of these nutrients are required to make T3 receptors inside the nucleus of our cells. If D and A are insufficient then the number or population of T3 receptors will be insufficient for the binding of T3. If T3 is plentiful but receptors are minimal then a person will experience hypothyroid symptoms.

The adrenal hormone cortisol is also involved. It primes these T3 receptor sites to optimize T3 binding. Cortisol can be checked through saliva hormone testing. If it is low then there are several means of improving levels including herbs, glandular extracts, plenty of rest, the maintenance of optimal blood sugar levels, a prescription for cortisol, and by increasing animal protein intake. A future section on cortisol will fill in the details.

You'll find a complete list of all the tests I've covered for each phase in a future chapter.

SECTION 4

BREAST DISEASE

"The only books that influence us are those for which we are ready,
and which have gone a little farther down
our particular path than we have yet got ourselves."

E.M. Forster

Breast & Thyroid Connection

There have been some amazing studies on breast disease published in medical journals over that last 60 years, some of which relate to Hashimoto's. But a little background on the relationship between breast cancer and thyroid hormones is important to start off with.

I feel there were two most important studies on breast cancer. One was published in *The Lancet* in 1976. It presented a global perspective, searching for answers to the question of why breast cancer was lower in some parts of the world than others. This investigation uncovered the fact that Japanese women had a much lower incidence of breast cancer than women living in the United States.

Examining cultural and lifestyle differences they discovered that the nutritional intake of iodine in the Japanese diet was about 15 times that of the U.S and very likely accounted for their lower incidence of breast disease. During that same period the hottest research was focused on the link between estrogen and breast cancer. The study hypothesized that iodine might help to metabolize or shift estrogens away from the estrone (E1) form towards estriol (E3). As a result of the *Lancet* study, our research into iodine and breast disease began.[44]

The other important study on breast cancer was done at the University of Pisa in Italy. They examined the relationship between breast cancer and thyroid disease using 102 women with ductal cell carcinoma. All had thyroid blood tests and thyroid ultrasounds.

The results were significant. Of the 102 women, 28 were diagnosed with nontoxic goiters, 16 with thyroid autoimmune disease, 2 with thyroid cancer and one with subacute thyroiditis, what I consider a pre-stage of Hashimoto's. That's a pretty significant figure, that just under half of them had a thyroid disease. I believe these numbers would have been significantly higher if the researchers had included women that suffered from Subclinical Hypothyroidism and suboptimal, or lower than optimal, hypothyroidism.

This study's conclusion focused solely on the recommendation that physicians treating women with breast cancer should also screen them for thyroid disease. But I believe the results uncovered something much more significant.[45]

Might these two studies hold the keys for preventing and possibly treating breast cancer?

Could it mean that the development of thyroid disease is a risk factor for breast disease?

Could it mean that the causes for a women developing nontoxic goiter, or thyroid autoimmune disease, or low thyroid hormones be the same causes behind the development of breast cancer?

Could it be that if we learn how to prevent and treat various thyroid diseases that we could also prevent and treat breast disease and breast cancer?

I believe the answer to all four of these questions is yes!

Breast Tissue

First let's examine what we know about breast tissue, the development of breast cancer and some of the known risk factors.

Breast cancer does not develop overnight. Breast tissue does not advance from healthy to malignant without passing through tissue changes such as dysplasia, cystic and fibrotic with pain and swelling. No matter how sophisticated our imaging technology has become in the detection of malignant growth, we still know that *benign* breast tissue changes increase the risk of breast cancer. The search for a cure for breast cancer must widen its focus to include prevention of these benign tissue changes. Unfortunately "the cure" is driven by research primarily supported by the ideal of a drug which targets cell receptors or genes, or a medical procedure. Research does not focus upon prevention or solutions that are not financially lucrative or patentable.

The general category for all breast tissue changes other than cancer is called benign breast disease (BBD). According to a 2005 article in the *New England Journal of Medicine*, BBD is a risk factor for developing breast cancer.[46]

Logically, then, to lower the incidence of breast cancer we need to treat and prevent BBD.

In 1997 the Ghent Report was submitted to the FDA. It was a double blind study involving 92 women with Fibrocystic Breast Disease which falls within the category of BBD. The women were treated with iodine with "significant improvement in breast tenderness, nodularity, fibrosis, turgidity, and the number of macrocysts."[47] The research clearly indicated a viable and effective treatment for benign breast disease. The Ghent Report was refused by the FDA, saying it could not endorse the trial since iodine is a natural substance and not a drug.

Another study published in *The Breast Journal* in 2004 involved 111 women with Cystic Mastalgia, painful breasts due to cysts. These selected participants had to have moderate to severe breast pain for six or more days each month. A significant improvement in breast pain, tenderness and breast nodularity was experienced within three months using 6 mg of iodine taken daily.[48]

I know this 6 mg dose is higher than I'm recommending but this research didn't investigate the long term effects of this dose, and didn't monitor thyroid antibodies. I'm sure that many people would be fine with this dose, but when I'm speaking to the general public I must remain conservative and be sure that my suggestions will do no harm.

Might it be a simple case that the higher intake of iodine in the Japanese women simply reduced the incidence of benign breast disease which lowered their risk of developing breast cancer? Could it be that simple? Let's hope so.

Now that you know that one of the underlying causes of developing thyroid inflammation, which increases the risk of developing Hashimoto's, is an iodide deficiency which is often accompanied by an iodine deficiency, might this not be one reason why women with Hashimoto's are at a higher risk for developing breast cancer?

NIS Channels

There is another quality about breast tissue that was recently discovered. For a long time, we knew that the absorption of iodide into the thyroid gland was through what's called the iodine trap, even though it traps iodide. Another name for this trap or channel is the sodium-iodide symport (NIS).

In the early 2000's we discovered that breast tissue also has these same NIS channels. Initially we thought these channels appeared only during the last trimester of pregnancy in order to supply iodine during lactation. Yet now we know that these same channels are found in the ductile cells of the breast, those cells most susceptible to breast cancer.[49]

We know that iodine helps to improve BBD and that breast tissue has specific NIS channels for iodine absorption. Knowing this brings up several concerns.

The first is that our National and Nutritional Surveys determined that 36 million people in the U.S. are iodine deficient.[50] This figure could easily be doubled it we included people with iodine *insufficiency.* Because of low iodine status, all these people are at risk for developing thyroid and breast disease.

The second concern is for those people diagnosed as hypothyroid and taking thyroid medication. When a person reaches this point of requiring a thyroid prescription they are very often severely iodine and iodide deficient. Research shows that people taking a thyroid prescription have an increased risk of developing breast disease.[51] Why would this be true?

I don't believe it has anything to do with the prescription but rather the underlying reason for why a person develops Hypothyroidism to the point of requiring a thyroid medication. Even though their prescription is helping to correct a deficiency of thyroid hormones, nothing has been done to address the cause, which is most often an iodide (iodine) deficiency.

A little side remark is needed here. In the 40's and 50's, when physicians discovered an epidemic of enlarged thyroids (goiter) we recognized that our female population was suffering from an iodide deficiency. Therefore iodized (iodide) salt was introduced as a way to remedy this, and for the most part it worked.

But no one asked why. Why would we suddenly have an iodide deficiency leading to an epidemic of thyroid goiter in specific regions of the United States?

Well, certainly it was because iodide was no longer available in high enough concentrations in our soils likely due to depletion and the changing practices in commercial agriculture.

But in nature seldom does iodide exist without its sister iodine. So yes, we did help to correct the iodide deficiency through the use of table salt but no one considered the body's need for iodine.

And another thought comes to mind. How many of us think that salt is bad for us. How many people are now avoiding salt because of the advice of their physician or subtle media propaganda?

Anyway, I do believe that we as a population are iodine and iodide deficient and we are suffering the consequences. Since our medical system thinks drugs and not nutrients or health we must, once again, become educated and take our health into our own hands.

The third concern I have is once again for the person taking a thyroid prescription. Taking Synthroid or L-thyroxin will cause a person's T4 levels to increase and their TSH to decline. In trying to help their patient feel better their physician will often increase the dose of thyroid medication to the point of causing their TSH to drop considerably. It is very important to keep TSH levels in an optimal range because this hormone stimulates the activity and the number of NIS channels in the thyroid, breast, ovaries and other tissues. Low levels of TSH, often occurring with thyroid medication, will indirectly reduce the uptake of iodine into these tissues.[52] [53] [54] Fortunately, for many people, taking iodine will increase TSH levels.

Breast Tissue & Estrogens

At puberty, normal breast tissue growth is primarily triggered by estrogens that bind to estrogen receptors on breast cells. Research in the 1970s discovered that malignant breast cell growth was stimulated by estrogens, if these cells had estrogen receptors. It was also discovered that the estrone (E1) form of estrogen binds to (stimulates) these cells five times longer than the other two forms, estradiol (E2) and estriol (E3).[55]

Most research has been directed towards estrogens and their receptors on breast cancer cells and very little towards estrogens and benign breast disease, even though BBD is a known risk factor. In 2008 the *Journal of the National Cancer Institute* disclosed a study showing that women taking estrogen have twice the risk of developing BBD. Their conclusion; "The prevailing hypothesis concerning the natural history (progression) of breast cancer is that benign proliferative breast disease…represents successive steps preceding the development of invasive breast [cancer]."[56] Again, we need to focus on prevention as well as treatment.

So now we know that estrogens are related to the development of BBD and we know that iodine improves BBD. The question then is how might iodine help to reduce the negative effects of estrogen?

Iodine

First let's look into some global statistics on breast cancer. I pulled out one study from a year before the *Lancet's* 1976 global cancer survey that I believe helps prove a point. Before the spread of international fast food chains, most people primarily ate food grown and raised locally. For this reason older studies may offer insights that since have become blurred by food importation and the relocation of populations.

I took a look at the growth of the largest fast food chain with the greatest influence on the eating habits of people around the world.

In 1948 McDonalds was founded. By 1958 it had sold 1,000,000 hamburgers ranging in price between 15 to 19 cents. By 1967 McDonalds opened in Canada and Puerto Rico. By 1978 the 5,000th McDonalds opened in Kanagawa, Japan. I am not saying or inferring that McDonald's hamburgers are the cause of higher rates of BBD or breast cancer in the United States, but I am trying to recognize the variable of substituting food from another culture which happened in Japan after the *Lancet* study.

In a 1975 article in *Health & Policy Planning* they also reviewed the international incidence of breast cancer. In North America there were approximately 105,300 women diagnosed with breast cancer, an average of 57 for every 100,000. That same year Japanese women had 11,500 with an average of 20 for every 100,000.[57] Some might say that we had better diagnostic technology and would thus show a higher incidence, but let's keep an open mind for a moment. We are trying to make discoveries and to learn ways of prevention. Later studies showed that Japanese women who relocated to the U.S. had an almost identical rate of breast cancer as women living in the United States.

Maybe iodine is the major factor and maybe it isn't. But as we go into this next section let us hypothesize for the moment that iodine is the primary means of preventing BBD and breast cancer.

Iodine Research

One method of researching a substance with suspected anti-carcinogenic effects is through animal studies. This often involves using genetically designed rats who respond to a specific carcinogen by developing the corresponding specific cancer. To test a substance's anti-carcinogenic ability, it is given simultaneously with the carcinogen to observe its effect in prevention or in delaying the onset of the cancer.

In 2001 a study used iodine in the form of an extract from seaweed to observe its protective effects against the carcinogen DMBA. Now where ever you find iodine in a food you will also find iodide.

The rats were placed in three groups. One group was fed commercial feed while the other two were fed the same feed mixed with differing amounts of the seaweed extract.

The conclusion was, "significant suppression of tumor growth was observed in groups 1-B and 1-C (seaweed mixed into feed) compared with 1-A (regular feed). These results suggest that iodine is transported through the serum into mammary tissues and induces apoptosis (death of cancer cells). Wakame (seaweed) suppressed the proliferation of DMBA induced mammary tumors."[58]

Their second study took a different route for the ingestion of the seaweed extract, "...extremely strong suppressive effect in rat mammary carcinogenesis when used in daily drinking water."[59]

Another study from 1996 expressed their results by stating, "The direct uptake of inorganic iodine by breast tumors led to the suppression of tumor growth."[60]

Another way that research can investigate a substance is through the use of human cell cultures. These studies are referred to as in vitro or outside the body. One study observed the effect of the seaweed extract on three kinds of human breast cancer cells. Again, the same apoptosis or cell death was observed. "These effects were stronger than those of chemotherapeutics widely used to treat human cancer cells."[61]

Even though these studies are very impressive it still remains unclear as to how iodine works.

Iodine & Estrogen

We've already covered the beneficial effects of iodine upon benign breast disease with one of the leading causes of BBD being high estrogens. So what is the link between estrogen and iodine's ability to counteract the stimulatory effects of estrogen?

Some believe that iodine shifts the concentration ratios of three estrogens (E1, E2 and E3) away from E1 towards E3. This would help since E1 stimulates breast cell receptors five times longer than

E2 or E3. Yet I could not find any research that proved this effect. All was hearsay and speculation.

However what has surfaced in the field of genetic research explains how iodine reduces the stimulatory effects of estrogens. I promise to keep this very simple.

Iodine and iodide alter the expression of several genes in the estrogen pathway. Iodine and iodide down regulate (quiet) several estrogen receptor genes, with the result being a slowing or repressing of estrogen's effects on breast cancer cell metabolism. This helps to explain the role of iodine in both prevention and treatment of BBD and breast cancer, when the breast cancer cells have estrogen receptors.

This research went one step further. Currently the one prescription used for the prevention and treatment of estrogen receptor positive breast cancer is Tamoxifen. How Tamoxifen works is not fully understood, but it's supposed to fit onto the estrogen receptor to block estrogen engagement. Yet this drug has the primary side effect of causing a drug resistant cancer because Tamoxifen stimulates a gene termed CCND1. As it turns out, their extensive study showed that iodine and iodide decrease CCND1 replication and thus enhances the effectiveness of Tamoxifen therapy.[62]

Thyroid Hormones

It looks like we've come full circle. To start at the beginning, let's examine the Pisa study for a moment and remember that 46% of the women with breast cancer suffered obvious thyroid disease.

Nontoxic goiter (NG) was the most pronounced. NG is caused by a combination of two things, low iodide and elevated estrogen. Elevated estrogens actually block the uptake of iodide into the thyroid cells <u>and</u> increases thyroid cell growth.[63] Research has shown that women with goiters have three times the incidence of breast cancer.[64]

The other major thyroid disease in the Pisa study was autoimmune thyroid disease. As we've already covered, the probable origin of AITD is an iodide deficiency. Research is now beginning to make another connection between AITD and breast cancer. There is evidence that people with AITD may also have antibodies that attack the NIS channels and thus decrease iodine uptake into the breast.[65] This evidence is not conclusive, yet another study remarked that "this inhibition of iodine uptake is due to unknown factors present in the sera (blood)" of Hashimoto's and Graves' patients.[66]

These two reasons, low iodide levels as the primary underlying cause of AITD, and the inhibition of iodine absorption into breast tissue seem like very plausible causes, or at least risk factors for AITD patients, to develop BBD and breast cancer.

Just recently, in 2008, the *Critical Review of Oncology and Hematology* published an article from the USC/Norris Comprehensive Cancer Clinic and the Keck School of Medicine at USC in Los Angeles, California. "We believe that the thyroid disease-breast cancer relationship provides a unique opportunity to find out the causes of breast cancer."[67]

They propose that the reduction of breast cancer in hyperthyroid patients, or patients with increased levels of thyroid hormones, is partly due to iodine which is driving biochemical mechanisms that generate apoptosis or the destruction of cancer cells.[68]

Another reason why plenty of thyroid hormones are important in the prevention of BBD and breast cancer is because thyroid hormones stimulate the production of sex hormone binding globulin known as SHBG.[69] SHBG is a protein that binds hormones, including estrogen. If SHBG goes down then more estrogens are free to leave the blood stream and to bind to estrogen receptors throughout the body including breast tissue. When thyroid hormones are low, as in hypothyroidism, then less SHBG is produced which leads to an increase in free estrogens.

Progesterone

A very simple study was performed by Linda Cowan and her team. From 1945 to 1965 a total of 1,083 women were evaluated and treated for infertility. These women were placed in 2 groups, the first one having infertility due to a progesterone deficiency and the second having non-hormonal causes. They were then followed through 1978 to determine the incidence of breast cancer.

Compared with the second group, the women with low progesterone had five times the rate of breast cancer. Cowan could not explain this higher rate to be anything other than low progesterone. Compared with controls, this progesterone deficiency group experienced a 10 fold increase in deaths from all malignant neoplasms.[70]

We know that the membranes of ovary cells have thyroid receptors. When thyroid hormones attach to these receptors they stimulate ovary cell activity. We also know that T3 stimulates ovary cells to convert pregnenalone into progesterone. Low T3 is one reason for low progesterone production.

Low levels of T3 often result from nontoxic goiter, thyroid autoimmune disease, and hypothyroidism. I believe that Cowan's research is another part of the puzzle, helping to confirm the relationship between thyroid disease and breast cancer since low thyroid hormones lead to low progesterone, which increases a woman's risk of developing breast cancer.[71]

Huff...Puff...

I know your head must be spinning by now. This chapter has taken me by far the longest time because of so many interconnections.

One last consideration is environmental carcinogens and their impact on breast tissue. Carcinogens have been in the public's mind for the last 30 years. The word carcinogen refers to any substance or particle that promotes cancer by inducing uncontrolled, malignant cell division and the formation of tumors.

In 1977 a journal showed how "Iodine deficient breast tissues are more susceptible to carcinogen action which promotes lesions earlier and in greater profusion."[72]

A study from Paris in 2008 identified "endocrine disrupting chemicals" (EDC) from cosmetics and pesticides leading to developmental defects and altered thyroid metabolism, with the major target of these chemicals being the NIS channels. This report confirmed that the negative effects of these chemicals were most pronounced in people with an iodine deficiency.

Summary

The WHO estimated 2 billion people in the world have an iodine deficiency and our National Health Survey estimated that 43 million Americans suffer the same. I believe we could double both these numbers if we also included those with an iodine insufficiency. And remember, as far as I am concerned, where there is an iodine deficiency there is also an iodide deficiency.

The world, and especially our nation, is suffering from obesity and a host of symptoms related to the multiple causes of low thyroid hormone symptoms, hormone deficiencies, BBD and cancers.

I truly believe that the prevention and treatment of BBD and breast cancer must integrate the use of iodine and iodide. We must educate the public about the prevention and treatment of Hashimoto's, and must comprehensively investigate the seven causes of low thyroid hormone symptoms and thyroid disease.

I believe that as we eliminate Hashimoto's and optimize thyroid hormone and levels of iodine and iodide, we will prevent millions of women from suffering the consequences of benign breast disease and breast cancer.

SECTION 5

CALL TO ACTION

"You can get help from teachers, but you are going to have to
learn a lot by yourself, sitting alone in a room."

Dr. Seuss

No One Will Ever Take Better Care of You than Yourself

Sometimes people wear their condition. There are the hand deformities of Rheumatoid Arthritis, the gait of Multiple Sclerosis and the discoloration and roughened skin of Psoriasis.

Hashimoto's is different because to outward appearance there are no distinguishing signs. Most people have never heard of Hashimoto's and when we try to explain our condition we often feel frustrated and confused.

Our lives shift the day we are diagnosed. We find ourselves in the grip of uncertainty, fear, anger, and loneliness.

Our physician often sidesteps our questions and offers vague remarks about Hashimoto's. Any questions are silenced by the remark, "There is no cure."

So now what? What's next?

It's true that the 1st step in treating Hashimoto's is the decision to take action. This first step is very personal and requires pure willpower and determination. It requires the realization that no one else can make this decision but you, and that no one can truly understand your needs better than you can.

Yet this does not mean that you must to do it alone. We all have the ability to create, and we are all pretty qualified when it comes to doing things alone. We can make things happen and we can accomplish, BUT we've also experienced what it's like to work with others in a harmonious group. We feel more alive, more motivated, and our energy and creativity are heightened. The human soul requires a frequent dose of community.

So as you read through this section, which covers the steps to take in treating Hashimoto's, remember that you don't have to do it alone.

Know the Use of Individual Lab Tests

First of all you know that you cannot treat Hashimoto's without lab results. If you have medical insurance they may cover some or all of the initial tests, YET some tests need repeating since we must monitor progress, to know when it's time to move from one phase of treatment to the next.

When insurance companies see a lab test repeated within a year they will often reject coverage and you will be billed. This can be extremely expensive. Many times people have compared what they paid their insurance company with what we charge. It was often five times more expensive. I am not saying you should use our services but if you can't get them where you live, we make them available. It may be that you order your tests through us yet continue to use your local physician.

Take a look at our website for lab testing costs.

Our goal is to share not only the information you need to steer your life towards greater health but to provide you with the tools for assessment along with an idea about how to understand lab results.

Here is how I think when it comes to interpreting lab results. This is based upon what physicians *should* know about the thyroid, on information found in medical research over the last 60 years, and upon what I've witnessed in practice.

A lot of this information can be found in current medical texts, yet unfortunately it's not in the mindset of most physicians. You may have already experienced the frustration of not having access to a knowledgeable physician, yet this book has been written to not only empower you, but to advance medical care from the grassroots up.

So let's set the premise that you have been diagnosed with Hashimoto's. What can you do next?

Ideally if money is not a concern then the following labs would be very helpful for navigating through Phases I & II. If finances are a consideration then TSH, T4 and the thyroid antibodies are most important. If previously you were positive for only one of the antibodies then just this one would need to be rechecked.

TSH	Thyroid stimulating hormone is very important. We need to keep it below 1.0 otherwise it will continue to stimulate H2O2 production in thyroid cells.
T4	This test reveals both the bound and Free T4. We need to know how well the thyroid is responding to TSH. If it's 8.0 and your TSH above 1.0 then the introduction of thyroid hormones will have to be very, very slow in order to decrease TSH below 1.0. I hope you understand that as we increase thyroid hormones with a prescription, TSH will come

down.

Free T4	This is the free form of T4 and helps to know how much of the T4 is bound and if there may be estrogen or liver issues. This is read always in relation to Total T4.
Free T3	This is the activating thyroid hormone. If this is low then we know one reason for low thyroid hormone symptoms. It is read or interpreted in relation to Free T4. If it's low we may need to improve thyroid hormone production, improve Free T4, assess cortisol levels, or use a T3 prescription.
Reverse T3	This may be elevated for a number of reasons. If it is, you should not use a prescription with T4 because it will likely form more Reverse T3. If Reverse T3 is elevated then the thyroid prescription must be T3 only.
TPO Antibodies	This tells us what levels of antibodies we are starting with and is used to monitor progress.
Anti-thyroglobulin Antibodies	This is another thyroid antibody, which is good to know about and, if elevated, will need to be monitored along with TPO.

Ferritin	This test assesses body stores of iron, with iron being one nutrient necessary for the thyroid to make its hormones. It is useful to know if iron needs to be supplemented in Phase I. Ideally ferritin should be around 60. If ferritin is higher than this you'll need to avoid iron in supplements.
Vitamin D	Vitamin D is required for the making of T3 nuclear receptor sites. Low vitamin D results in a lowered binding of T3 with the person having low thyroid symptoms. Ideally, vitamin D should be around 60.
Fasting glucose	Low blood sugar complicates and accentuates the symptoms of Hashimoto's. Fluctuating blood sugar levels including low blood sugar or hypoglycemia stress the adrenals and immune system. Ideally fasting glucose should be around 90.
Liver Enzymes	The AST and ALT are liver enzymes and if elevated can be one reason for bound T4 and poor conversion of T4 to T3.
Complete Blood	This includes the number of red blood cells,

Count (CBC)	the amount of hemoglobin inside these cells and the red blood cell volume. If there is anemia or a low red blood cell count then the body's lack of oxygen will hamper recovery. The CBC also includes the white blood cell count. This is a general way to assess lowered resistance to infection and the possibility of either an acute or a chronic silent infection.
Cholesterol & Other Fats	Cholesterol is essential for the body to make its various hormones including vitamin D. The optimal level of cholesterol is around 180.
Estradiol (saliva)	This is important to know about especially in relation to progesterone.
Progesterone (saliva)	Checking progesterone in relation to estradiol is always important. Remember that progesterone stimulates receptors on thyroid cells.
Cortisol (saliva)	Readings for both am and pm are important for knowing if low cortisol might be one reason for poor T4 to T3 conversion. This hormone is also involved with priming T3 nuclear receptor sites inside cells, and low

levels are associated with fatigue.

So, looking over a report with all these values I usually first cover deficiencies or insufficiencies. Here's what I would consider from the above. We'll cover thyroid hormones in a moment.

Vitamin D	Optimal is 60 so I'd start supplementing anyone below 40. Typical doses would be between 2,500 IU and 10,000 IU depending upon how low their reading is. If a person supplements, I suggest checking vitamin D again in 3 months. Certainly sunlight is the best way to increase vitamin D levels and usually a half hour a day in a swimsuit is ideal. Remember that for the body to make vitamin D, cholesterol is required.
Cholesterol	Ideally it should be around 180. If it is higher than 200 it may be due to low thyroid hormones. Elevated cholesterol is often a sign of hypothyroidism. If it's less than 160 I suggest increasing animal protein intake.
Estradiol	I like to see this at 2.0 or less on a saliva hormone test, but this hormone must always be evaluated in relation to progesterone.

Higher than 2.0 may warrant some cleansing of the liver using a variety of herbs including milk thistle. High estradiol is often due to poor metabolism or breakdown of this hormone, which takes place in the liver. Remember that the major source of non-endocrine estrogen production is fat cells. Extra weight can lead to elevated estrogens.

Progesterone	This is very often low. I like to see a minimum of 100 on a saliva hormone test. Low progesterone can be due to low thyroid hormone stimulation of the ovaries, low cholesterol, and stress. It may be useful to temporarily use either a prescription of progesterone or Emerita's 'natural' Pro-Gest cream listed on our site. If you have headaches or difficulty staying asleep then capsules may be the best form. Best to recheck estrogen and progesterone hormones about 3-6 months later.
Cortisol	Cortisol is highest in the mornings and will decline through the day. It's best to check morning saliva and again before bed. This

gives a pretty good idea about the strength of the adrenals and their ability to sustain cortisol levels throughout the day. I like to see cortisol in the 20's in the am and around 2 before bed. Low levels of cortisol are important to correct when treating immune problems. Cortisol is improved with B vitamins, especially B5, and magnesium, by maintaining optimal blood sugar levels, and plenty of sleep and rest with a bare minimum of 8 hours a night.

Low Red Blood Cell Count	Anemia has several causes and the CBC test will help determine if it's due to iron and B12. Usually supplementation is essential. B12 should be taken sublingually to be absorbed well. Taking 2 mgs is usually adequate and is taken with folic acid. For iron deficiency anemia you may be able to use an herbal preparation, unless your ferritin is low.
Ferritin	Ideally this is around 60-70. If it is below 25 then I suggest using a product called Ferritin from Cardiovascular Research. Otherwise using iron in various forms is fine. Taking vitamin C with meals with help to absorb

more iron from your food.

If it is above 100 then never use a supplement with iron. It it's above 200 you need to investigate ways of lowering it. High ferritin is a risk factor for cardiac and other problems.

Fasting Glucose   Ideally fasting blood sugar should be between 85 and 95. If it's less than 85 then there's a tendency to low blood sugar or hypoglycemia. This puts stress on the adrenals, adding to fatigue and fluctuating blood sugar levels. Using chromium at 200mcg will improve this, but it's important to stay away from sugars and simple carbohydrates. I've already mentioned the importance of animal protein and the avoidance of high glycemic foods for controlling blood sugar problems.

So that's about it for all the non-thyroid tests. Now let's look at the thyroid and thyroid antibodies.

The first objective with treating Hashimoto's is to get TSH below 1.0 (mIU/ml).

If it is above 1.0, and your thyroid hormone T4 is below 7.5 (ug/dL), then you can use a little compounded T4 and T3 depending upon a few things. The level of 7.5 is pretty close to the optimum of 8.5 so you don't need much. If T4 is below 7.5, then of course you can use a little more, but the way of taking the thyroid medication still applies, which is to start slowly and work your way up based on monitoring your heart rate and your overall symptoms.

We've got to get your T4 up enough to slow down the production of TSH.

I have likely mentioned this in another section but it bears repeating. When you first start taking a thyroid prescription, or any time you increase your thyroid hormone intake, you are going to feel better. But with this increase, your TSH will decline and your own endogenous production of thyroid hormones will decline as well. This will feel like two steps forward and one step back. This will happen and I hope you understand why.

If your Free T3 level is in the midrange (look at the lab's reference range and find the midpoint) then you likely don't need T3 added to your compounded T4 and T3 prescription. If your Free T3 is less than optimal then add T3 to your prescription.

Synthroid and L-thyroxin are measured in milligrams. Thyroid glandulars are also measured in milligrams and also grains. Compounded thyroid medication is measured in micrograms.

A 60mg prescription of either Synthroid or a glandular is equivalent to about 38mcg of T4 and 9mcg of T3 of the compounded form. You want to start at about a third of this, which is around 13mcg of T4 and 3mcg of T3. This is the place to start for the first 7-10 days. Then increase by the same amount each 7-10 days until you've found what dose feels best and may increase heart rate just a little.

If your TSH is below 1.0 and your Total T4 is optimal (around 8.0 to 8.5) then you really don't need to take a T4 prescription. If your TSH is above 1.0 and your Total T4 is optimal you'll still need to take some T4 in very small increments to get your TSH below 1.0.

If your Free T3 is on the low side then add some T3 to the prescription. You can start with about 2.5 mcg twice daily about 10-12 hours apart. This is a starting dose and can be increased every four to seven days if needed.

If Total T4 is optimal but Free T4 (ng/dL) is suboptimal, then you need to look at getting estrogen lowered and progesterone improved, and also some liver cleansing. Since your thyroid hormone production (T4) is OK I do not suggest using a thyroid prescription unless your TSH is above 1.0.

You'll learn more about follow-up lab testing a little further on.

If you are already taking a thyroid medication all the above still applies. It may just be a matter of tweaking what you are already taking and adding some T3.

If Reverse T3 is elevated and your Total T4 is optimal (8.0 to 8.5) then you cannot take a thyroid prescription that includes T4 because it will likely cause even more Reverse T3 to be made. Reverse T3 is made from T4. Very often when Reverse T3 is high Free T3 will be low. Therefore the approach is to use a T3 prescription. This will improve your energy and help to reduce Reverse T3. When you are increasing your T3 medication it is important to monitor both heart rate and body temperature. Increased heart rate will tell you if you are taking too much and an increase in body temperature will tell you that your body is responding by increasing its metabolic rate. Best time to take your temperature is first thing in the morning. This is known as your basal body temperature.

On our site you'll find a listing of all the above tests.

Phase II Lab Testing

You enter Phase II when your thyroid antibodies are within normal limits.

In Phase II, the primary goal is to increase your thyroid's production of thyroid hormones without causing an increase of thyroid antibodies. This increase is achieved by introducing iodine and iodide while continuing to take all the nutrients the thyroid requires to make its hormones. During this second phase we must monitor thyroid antibodies and TSH.

TSH will most likely rise with the introduction of iodine and iodide, but this increase will not necessarily lead to thyroid inflammation since there's plenty of circulating glutathione and selenium.

Once you've been on 3 mg of iodine and iodide for two weeks it's time to recheck thyroid antibodies. If these are still normal then we need to do a complete thyroid lab panel. This is to know how well your thyroid is working and if there are any problems with converting T4 to T3.

Sometimes the thyroid is able to produce optimal levels of thyroid hormones and sometimes not. To a large degree this depends upon how much thyroid damage was caused by the inflammation.

Here are the tests to perform if your thyroid antibodies remained normal.

- ~ TSH- I know this test was recently done but when checking thyroid hormones a single draw is important when checking all thyroid hormone values. We need to be sure that your thyroid is getting the stimulation it needs to make its hormones. We also want to know how well your pituitary is responding to the iodide and iodine. TSH is one way to assess that.
- ~ T4
- ~ Free T4
- ~ Free T3

If your Reverse T3 was elevated then this needs to be repeated.

You should have a pretty good idea by now about interpreting these tests and what needs to be done to tweak or optimize their levels. If you need more help then I suggest reading *Low Thyroid Hormone Symptoms- 7 Causes & 7 Solutions*, my first book.

"With every experience, you alone are painting your own canvas,

thought by thought, choice by choice."

Oprah Winfrey

Restore Your Health Day-by-Day & Step-by-Step

Just to add some clarity, here are the steps for each phase.

Phase I

The five primary goals of this phase are the following;

1. Reduce thyroid inflammation by lowering TSH

2. Reduce thyroid inflammation through supplements and a gluten free diet

3. Nourish the thyroid gland in preparation for Phase II

4. Repair thyroid cells through supplements

5. Treat other contributing conditions, such as Candida, mold allergies and heavy metals

1) Reduce thyroid inflammation by lowering TSH

~ Thyroid medication increased in small increments

~ Avoid iodine and iodide in supplements and in food

2) Reduce thyroid inflammation through supplements

~ Selenium methionine 400mcg for increasing glutathione

~ N-Acetyl Cysteine at 1,000mg twice daily to increase glutathione production

~ Sublingual L-Glutathione 150mg dissolved twice daily under the tongue

~ Topical DMSO with glutathione applied 2-3 times daily over the thyroid

~ Omega III taking 2,000 IU a day with food

~ Just a reminder about kicking the gluten habit

3) Nourish the thyroid gland in preparation for Phase II

~ Selenium methionine but not more than 400mcg daily

~ Zinc picolinate 25-50mg taken once daily

~ Iron, if your Ferritin blood test is less than 40. Take between 20-30mg per day of the product Ferritin, with food.

~ Vitamin A, preferably in the mycellized form at 30,000 IUs. This dose is too high for pregnant women and should be reduced to below 10,000 IUs.

~ Essential Fatty Acids, preferably with fish, flax and borage seed oils. (Optimal EFA's)

~ ATP CoFactors, take one, twice daily. This is B2 at 100mg and B3 as inositol hexanicotinate at 500mg

4) Repair thyroid cells through supplements

~ Mixed EFA's from Biotics Research. It contains Walnut, Hazelnut, Sesame, and Apricot Kernel oils.

5) Treat other underlying conditions which affect Hashimoto's

~ Candida and improving gut ecology

~ Colostrum Plus from Symbiotics but there are others

~ Acidophilus after the Colostrum (Bacillus Coagulans)

~ Grapefruit Seed Extract (GSE) in capsule and liquid form

~ SF722 Thorne Research taken after the GSE

~ Tanalbit taken after the SF722.

~ Remember the Candida nutritional part of the program.

If you have a mold allergy then...

~ Bio-Aller Mold, Dust and Yeast

~ Stinging Nettles or Uva Ursi for some immediate relief

~ Clean up your environment of molds

For heavy metal detoxification the N-Acetyl Cysteine helps but also consider...

~ Waiora liquid

Phase II

~ Lugol's 2%

~ Continue with all the supplements from Phase I.

Phase III

~ All the supplements for optimizing thyroid hormone production based upon thyroid and other lab tests performed at the end of Phase II.

~ Continue with all the supplements from Phase I and II. You are really home free, and now it's a matter of continued improvement and maintenance.

Whenever a person has had a condition, they will always be prone to a reoccurrence. I do believe that by maintaining the supplements and the nutritional guidelines, the chance of Hashimoto's coming back is pretty slim.

"It is our choices, Harry, that show what we truly are,

far more than our abilities."

J. K. Rowling

Reflections

Before we go on to 'Resources' in the next section, it's important to mention something.

In that first month of research, gathering every journal article I could find on the subjects of thyroid inflammation and Hashimoto's, I remember sitting at a table in the medical school library with several stacks of around 200 articles and entries from medical texts.

I felt overwhelmed, adrift in a sea of information, not knowing how to piece it all together. I sensed the destination, of finding the cause of Hashimoto's, but how would I get there? Each stack was a different medical perspective yet no one, as far as I could tell, had found the common link.

There were dark periods of doubt. Who was I to think that I could find the key? Studies and facts raced through my mind seemingly disconnected and random without an anchor.

I thought of Einstein and how in the end, after years of speculation, theory and creative imagination, he synthesized his work down to a simple explanation, $E=mc^2$.

Finally clarity arrived, that the step prior to Hashimoto's was thyroid inflammation and… well, you know the rest.

This research was then applied and put into practice with the expected results.

Then the book began for two reasons.

The first was to provide the research in a simple, easily understood form with relative ease of application by anyone with Hashimoto's.

The second reason was to indirectly inform and influence physicians, to present the research on pharmacy and nutrients, and how it could be integrated into clinical practice.

Generally, it was a desire to advance the quality and effectiveness of care for Hashimoto's.

Yet near the middle of the book I began to think, what good is this information for people with Hashimoto's if they cannot apply it, if they cannot put it into practice, if they cannot find a cooperative physician?

After a conversation with my daughter, Justyn, we agreed to provide everything a person needs for treatment. We both knew that by including this we were stepping out on a limb for a number of reasons. There are many laws regulating the practice of medicine. There are strong forces which promote and financially support the pharmaceutical approach to treating every condition.

The point is that the primary intent of writing this book was not to sell services, labs and supplements. I simply want to clarify this because we have all become so sensitive and cynical about the ulterior intentions of other, that their motive is to sell us something... again!

But where is the integrity of selling something to someone without truly understanding the needs of that someone.

So again, the primary intention is not to sell you something. We have given you everything you need to do this on your own locally, with the cooperation of your physician, where you live.

Now, if you intend to work with your physician I doubt if he or she will have an interest in reading this book, especially since I am a Naturopathic Physician. They would much prefer to see the science and research.

We therefore compiled a 115 page pdf document for physicians. It contains the word-for-word abstracts from all the medical research journals and medical texts that were referenced in both *Hope for Hashimoto's* and *Low Thyroid Hormones- 7 Causes & 7 Solutions*. The table of contents makes it super easy to search through.

I am sure that in this format your physician would take an interest, which would foster a more educated and receptive relationship between the two of you.

To receive this document, simply submit your request to advancingcare@gmail.com.

Our intention, once again, is to help you to improve your condition by providing whatever you need and this includes helping you to find your medical support locally.

One question we are often asked is, do we know of a physician in their city whom we can refer. Right now, we don't but we are hoping this will change in the near future.

This next section on resources we'll briefly describe some of the services and products we offer.

"With the new day comes new strength and new thoughts."

Eleanor Roosevelt

Resources

I would like to say that you can recover from Hashimoto's. I have seen it and I know it's possible. Yet I also know it's impossible to predict who will and who won't. I can say though, that I am certain that you will feel better when following the guidelines.

You can supply the nutrients your body needs to reduce inflammation.

You can remove specific foods from your diet giving you more energy and better concentration.

You can use thyroid medication to optimize thyroid hormone levels without any side effects.

You can improve the ecology of the gut which will improve many of your symptoms.

You can saturate your body with iodine and iodide for protecting against endocrine disrupting chemicals and the prevention of other more severe conditions.

You can optimize thyroid hormone production, metabolism and utilization using natural methods.

I know this amount of information can feel overwhelming, especially if you are feeling tired both physically and mentally but an education is the key to success.

I know that very often this path to recovery can feel a little lonely, yet you are not alone. We are here to help.

Prescriptions

You will likely need a prescription if you are not already taking one. And if you are taking the synthetic thyroid hormone (Synthroid or levothyroxine) you can add Cytomel or T3. Or you might switch to a compounded T4 and T3. In any case you can approach your physician for a prescription.

You also have the option of scheduling a 30 minute consultation with either a licensed physician on our staff or myself. We can then take care of the prescription. If you have a Naturopathic Physician nearby, they may also be able to help.

We also use a couple of compounding pharmacies that will even ship overseas.

Again, as a reminder, acupuncture and homeopathy can accelerate recovering your health but your primary provider must be able to provide the necessary lab tests and the prescriptions.

Lab Testing Services

We do provide blood lab testing for clients in the United States and it's relatively painless (that was a joke).

For blood work, once it is paid for, we simply mail your LabCorp requisition to you. This requisition is taken to any LabCorp Patient Service Center in your city. To check if there's a Center nearby go to www.labcorp.com, click 'find a lab' and enter your zip code. This service is unavailable in NY, RI, and NJ because of state restrictions.

Your results are emailed to us usually within three days after the blood draw and they will be immediately forwarded to you. Be sure to include your email address when completing the form in our shopping cart.

Seldom will an MD agree with using saliva hormone testing. You can learn more about the accuracy of this method by visiting the site www.labrix.com. Saliva hormone kits are mailed to your home address. You then return the kit directly to the lab. The same restrictions apply for NY, RI and NJ.

These saliva kits can be shipped overseas but you'll need to contact our office since shipping and handling costs vary from one country to the next.

Storefront

We provide all supplements through our estore on Amazon. They provide great inventory and shipping services.

The purchase of lab tests and ebooks is through One Shopping Cart. Further details about our storefront can be found on our site.

Consultations

Information on consultations is under dropdown 'Services' on our site. We provide information packets that explain the details of this service. One packet is for those living in the United States and the other for those living outside the U.S.

"We delight in the beauty of the butterfly
but rarely admit the changes it has gone through
to achieve that beauty."

Maya Angelou

Final Words

I hope you've found much more than what you were searching for. When we launched this project of Hope for Hashimoto's we could only imagine the scope and breadth of where it would lead us. To say the least, we are filled with enthusiasm, about transmitting this message of hope around the world. We believe that everyone should have access to health care, to labs, prescriptions, and supplements.

We ask that you become involved in your recovery, as well as helping others. Assisting others can include sharing this information with friends and family as well as making comments on various community sites.

If you know someone with thyroid issues or symptoms, encourage them to be checked for Hashimoto's. Most physicians do not order labs for Hashimoto's because whether their patient has Hypothyroidism or Hashimoto's, their approach to treatment is the same.

Remember, the most common cause of Hypothyroidism is Hashimoto's. If it turns out that they don't have Hashimoto's then suggest they read *Low Thyroid Hormone Symptoms- 7 Causes and 7 Solutions.* It explains how and why a person with low thyroid hormones is seldom diagnosed properly. The softcover is listed on Amazon and the ebook is found on our site.

Through the use of today's technology we can leverage our influence and the advancement of Hashimoto's and thyroid care.

Before closing this book make a wish. Take a few moments to consider this.

What is it I wish for?

And now ask...

What single, simple action can I take right now, this very moment, that would help carry me one step closer to my wish?

All that's required is desire, some determination, a little help, and for some, a leap of faith.

Thanks,

Dr. Alexander Haskell, N.D.

www.HopeForHashimotos.com

"You gain strength, courage and confidence by every experience in which you really stop to look fear in the face. You are able to say to yourself, 'I have lived through this horror. I can take the next thing that comes along.' You must do the thing you think you cannot do."

Eleanor Roosevelt

Some people care too much, I think it's called love.

Winnie the Pooh

"I will not play tug o' war. I'd rather play hug o' war where everyone hugs instead of tugs, where everyone giggles and rolls on the rug, where everyone kisses and everyone grins, and everyone cuddles and everyone wins."

Shel Silverstein

"If you want something said, ask a man; if you want something done, ask a woman."

Margaret Thatcher

Those who dance are considered insane by those who cannot hear the music.

George Carlin

INDEX

A

Adrenal Fatigue, 24, 116

Allergies, 124

   Mold, 124

B

Blood Sugar

   Glycemic Index of Foods, 131

   Hashimoto's, 129

Breast Cancer

   Benign Breast Disease, 182

   Comparison US & Japan, 189

   Fibrocystic Breast Disease, 182

   Iodine & Estrogens, 191

   Iodine Research, 189

   Progesterone, 195

   Thyroid Disease, 194

Breast Disease

   Estrogens, 187

   Global Perspective, 179

   Hashimoto's, 179, 180

   Iodine, 183, 188

   NIS Channels, 184

   Sex Hormone Binding Globulin, 194

   Thyroid Hormones, 193

C

Candida, 133

   Books, 135

   Diet, 138

   Four-fold Approach, 135

   Product Recommendations, 136

   Symptoms, 134

Celiac Disease, 112

   Autoimmune Thyroid Disease, 113

   Selenium Deficiency, 113

Cholesterol, 142

   Female Hormones, 143

Cortisol, 116

Cortisone, 119

Cytozyme AD, 122

D

Dr. William Jefferies, M.D., 118

E

Endocrine Disrupting Chemicals, 45

Essential Fatty Acids, 107

G

Glutathione

    Sublingual, 110

Gluten Intolerrance, 112

H

Halogens, 150

Hashimoto's

    Breast Disease, 179

    Most common Rx, 33

Heavy Metals, 151

    Chelation, 155

    Chelation Waiora, 157

    Glutathione, 151

    Holistic Dentist, 152

    Mercury, 152

Hydrogen Peroxide

    Iodide to Iodine, 40

Hypothyroidism

    Primary & Secondary, 83

I

Inflammation of Thyroid

    Extinguish the Flame, 108

    Reduce TSH, 94

Iodine

    & Hashimoto's, 44

    Dangers, 70

    Deficiency in US, 184

    Diluting Lugol's, 166

    Elevated TSH, 71

    Incremental Dosing, 165

    Lugol's, 166

    Necessary for Health, 76

    Reduction of Breast Cancer, 47

    Reintroduction, 164

    Sodium Iodide Symports, 77

    Table for # of Tablespoons, 168

Iron

    Testing, 107

L

Lab Testing

    Necessity of, 81

M

Mercury
  Chelation, 155
  Chelation Waiora, 157
  Environmental Protection
    Agency, 154
  Holistic Dentist, 152
  Holistic Dentistry, 155
  Safe Ingestion?, 154
Molds, 125

N

N Acetyl Cysteine
  Dosage, 110

O

Ozone
  Molds, 128

P

Pantothenic Acid, 121

R

Reverse T3, 87

S

Safe Uses of Cortisol, 118
Selenium
  Antibody Reduction, 109
  Deficiency with Celiac Disease, 113
  Dosage, 107
  Production of Glutathione, 109
  Reduced Antibodies by 76%, 110
  Reducing Hydrogen Peroxide, 109
  Thyroid Cell Protection, 108
Sodium Iodide Symports, 77

T

Thyroid
  Essential Nutrients, 106
Thyroid Hormones
  Balancing, 173
  Lab Tests, 173
  Prescribing for Hashimoto's, 87
  T3, 57
  T3 half-life, 100
  T4 half-life, 86
  TSH half-life, 88
Thyroid Prescription, 53

Incremental Dosing, 100

Synthroid & Levothyroxine, 66

Thyroperoxidase, 42

TSH, 38

Helps to store iodine, 45

V

Vitamin A

Dosage, 107

Vitamins B2 & B3

Dosage, 107

W

Waiora, 157

Z

Zinc

Dosage, 107

REFERENCES

[1] Current Opinions in Endocrinology, Diabetes and Obesity. 2007 Jun14(3):197-208

[2] Rev Med Chil. 2010 Jan;138(1):15-21. Epub 2010 Mar 26.

[3] *Physiology* Mosby Press 4th Edition 1998 p. 912

[4] *Physiology* Mosby Press 4th Edition 1998 p.914

[5] *Physiology* Mosby Press 4th Edition 1998 p.913

[6] *Physiology* Mosby Press 4th Edition 1998 p.913

[7] Journal of Endocrinology. 2005 Mar;184(3):455-65.

[8] Hellenic Journal of Nuclear Medicine. 2007 Jan-Apr;10(1):6-8.

[9] Exp Biol Med (Maywood). 2010 Apr 1;235(4):424-33.

[10] Antioxid Redox Signal. 2008 Sep;10(9):1577-92.

[11] J Clin Endocrinol Metab. 2007 Oct;92(10):3764-73. Epub 2007 Jul 31.

[12] Endocr Relat Cancer. 2009 Sep;16(3):845-56. Epub 2009 Jun 9.

[13] Nature 459, 996-999 (18 June 2009)

[14] Best Pract Res Clin Endocrinol Metab. 2010 Feb;24(1):13-27.

[15] Endocr J. 2008 Dec;55(6):1103-8. Epub 2008 Aug 9.

[16] Eur J Endocrinol. 2008 Feb;158(2):209-15.

[17] Clin Endocrinol (Oxf). 2008 Jul;69(1):136-41. Epub 2008 Jul 1.

[18] Best Pract Res Clin Endocrinol Metab. 2010 Feb;24(1):13-27.

[19] Endocr J. 2008 Dec;55(6):1103-8. Epub 2008 Aug 9.

[20] Eur J Endocrinol. 2008 Feb;158(2):209-15.

[21] Clin Endocrinol (Oxf). 2008 Jul;69(1):136-41. Epub 2008 Jul 1.

[22] Journal of Endocrinology & Metabolism. 2001 Vol.86, No.10:4585-4590

[23] *Physiology* Mosby Press 4th Edition 1998 p.912

[24] Endocr J. 2008 Dec;55(6):1103-8

[25] Best Pract Res Clin Endocrinol Metab. 2010 Feb;24(1):107-15.

[26] Nat Clin Pract Endocrinol Metab. 2008 Aug;4(8):454-60. Epub 2008 Jul 8.

[27] Biol Chem. 2007 Oct;388(10):1053-9.

[28] Thyroid. 2006 May;16(5):455-60.

[29] J Endocrinol. 2005 Mar;184(3):455-65.

[30] Biol Chem. 2007 Oct;388(10):1053-9.

[31] Clin Endocrinol (Oxf). 2009 Dec 18. [Epub ahead of print]

[32] Best Pract Res Clin Endocrinol Metab. 2009 Dec;23(6):815-27.

[33] Antioxid Redox Signal. 2008 Sep;10(9):1577-92.

[34] Biofactors. 2003;19(3-4):121-30

[35] Thyroid. 2006 May;16(5):455-60

[36] Journal of Endocrinology. 2005 Mar;184(3):455-65.

[37] Eur J Endocrinol. 2003 Apr;148(4):389-93.

[38] Endocrinology Review. 2005 Dec;26(7):944-84.

[39] Biological Trace Element Research. 2008 Dec;126(1-3).

[40] Endocrine Practice. 2008 Apr;14(3):381-8.

[41] Journal of Pediatrics. 2009 Jul'155(1):51-5.
[42] Minerva Med.2008 Dec;99(6):643-53.
[43] Eur J Endocrinol. 2003 Apr;148(4):389-93.
[44] Lancet. 1976 Apr 24;1(7965):890-1.
[45] Journal of Clinical Endocrinology & Metabolism. 1996; 81:990-994.
[46] New England Journal of Medicine. 2005 Jul 21;353(3):229-37.
[47] Extrathyroidal Benefits of Iodine. Dr. Donald W. Miller,Jr.,M.D.,www.jpans.org
[48] The Breast Journal. 2004; 10(4);328-336
[49] Medicina 1997;57(Suppl 2):81-91.
[50] Journal of Clinical Endocrinology & Metabolism. 1998 Oct;83(10):3401-8.
[51] *Physiology* Mosby Press 4th Edition 1998 p.912
[52] Molecular Endocrinology. 2006 May;20(5):1121-37.
[53] Endocrine Reviews. 2003;24(1):48-77.
[54] Journal of Biological chemistry 2001;276(24):21458-63.
[55] Endocrinology. 1980;106(2):434-439.
[56] Journal of the National Cancer Institute. 2008; Apr100:519
[57] Health & Policy Planning. 1975;5(1): 1-22.
[58] Japan Journal Cancer Research. 1999 Sep;90(9):922-7.
[59] Japan Journal Cancer Research. 2001 May;92:483-7.
[60] Journal of Surgical Oncology. 1996 Mar;61(3):209-13.
[61] Japan Journal Cancer Research. 2001 May;92:483-7.
[62] International Journal of Medical Sciences. 2008; 5:189-196.
[63] Endocrine Reviews. 2003;24(1):48-77.
[64] Cancer Causes & Control. 2000; 11:121-127.
[65] European Journal of Endocrinology. 2006; 155(4):495-512.
[66] Endocrine Reviews. 2003; 24(1):48-77.
[67] Critical Reviews in Oncology/Hematology. 2008 Nov;68(2):107-14.
[68] Ibid.
[69] *Physiology* Mosby Press 4th Edition 1998 p.983.
[70] American Journal of Epidemiology. 1981;114(2):209-217.
[71] Endocrine Regulations. 1999;33:155-60.
[72] Advances in Experimental Medicine & Biology. 1977; 91:293-304

Notes

CPSIA information can be obtained at www.ICGtesting.com
Printed in the USA
BVOW021122160613

323434BV00014B/203/P